The
# Infertility
## Survival Handbook

# The
# Infertility
## Survival Handbook

■

EVERYTHING YOU NEVER THOUGHT
YOU'D NEED TO KNOW

## Elizabeth Swire Falker

Riverhead Books
New York

RIVERHEAD BOOKS
Published by The Berkley Publishing Group
A division of Penguin Group (USA) Inc.
375 Hudson Street
New York, New York 10014

Copyright © 2004 by Elizabeth Swire Falker
Book design by Tiffany Estreicher
Cover design by Claire Vaccaro

First Riverhead edition: April 2004

Library of Congress Cataloging-in-Publication Data

Falker, Elizabeth Swire.
    The infertility survival handbook : everything you never thought you'd need to know / Elizabeth Swire Falker.
        p.   cm.
    Includes bibliographical references and index.
    ISBN 1-57322-381-6
    1. Infertility—Handbooks, manuals, etc.   2. Fertility, Human—Handbooks, manuals, etc.
3. Human reproductive technology—Handbooks, manuals, etc.   I. Title.

RC889.F355   2004
618.1'78—dc22

                                                                                            2003067462

Printed in the United States of America

10   9   8   7   6   5   4   3   2   1

*For David,*
*who fills my heart and soul with joy.*
*I am honored to be your mother.*

# Contents

*Foreword* ................................................................. xi

*Acknowledgments* ....................................................... xiii

*Introduction: Acknowledging That Infertility Sucks!*
*Oh Baby, Does It Suck!* ............................................... xv


1. Telling My Story ..................................................... 1
THE GOOD, THE BAD, AND THE INSPIRATIONAL


2. Surviving the Infertility Roller Coaster ..................... 23
THIS DEFINITELY AIN'T A VACATION AT DISNEY WORLD


3. Finding a Good Reproductive
Endocrinologist or Fertility Clinic .......................... 30
YOU BETTER LIKE YOUR DOCTOR, BECAUSE YOU'RE ABOUT TO BUY HER A NEW BMW

Making Sense of Success Rates 48


4. Testing, Testing, Testing! ..................................... 55
FINDING OUT WHAT'S GOING ON AND WHAT'S GOING WRONG

Blood Tests 56 • Serum Progesterone Blood Test 56 • FSH, LH, and Estradiol Blood
Tests 56 • Prolactin and Androgen Blood Tests 57 • Genetic Testing for IVF Failure
and Recurrent Pregnancy Loss 58 • Immune Testing for IVF Failure and Recurrent
Pregnancy Loss 59 • Tests for Blood-Clotting Disorders 60 • Tests for Antibody Problems 61 • Tests for Baby-Killing Cells 63 • More Invasive Tests 64 • Endometrial

Biopsy 65 • Hysterosalpinogram (HSG) 67 • Saline Sonogram or Saline HSG 69 • Hysteroscopy 70 • Laparoscopy 71

5. Getting Your Diagnosis ........................................ 73
WHAT'S WRONG WITH ME?

Endometriosis 73 • Fallopian Tubes and Other Structural Problems 77 • Fibroids and Polyps 80 • Luteal Phase Defect (LPD) 83 • Polycystic Ovarian Syndrome (PCO, PCOS, Stein-Leventhal Syndrome, Syndrome X, and Syndrome O) 84 • Premature Ovarian Failure, High FSH, and Poor Responders 88 • Recurrent Pregnancy Loss and IVF Failure 93 • Blood-Clotting Disorders 93 • The Baby-Killing Cells 95 • Unexplained Infertility 97

6. Calling All Men ................................................. 99
YES, INFERTILITY AFFECTS MEN, TOO

Urologists and Semen Analyses 100 • ICSI (Intracytoplasmic Sperm Injection) 106 • Anatomical Issues That Cause Problems with Sperm Production 107 • Varicoceles 107 • Congenital Absence of the Vas Deferens 108 • Hypospadias 109 • Retrograde Ejaculation 109 • Other Anatomical Problems Caused by Blockages in the Reproductive Tract Due to Infection or from a Vasectomy 109 • Surgery and Azoospermia 110 • Supporting the Infertile Man 113

7. Deciding Which Family-Building
Option Is Best for You ........................................ 117
IT'S ALL A QUESTION OF NEEDLES

Adoption 119 • Alternative Therapies 125 • Child-Free Living 127 • Egg and Sperm Donation 128 • Embryo Donation 131 • Intrauterine Insemination 132 • In Vitro Fertilization 134 • GIFT (Gamete Intrafallopian Transfer) 137 • Natural Cycle IVF 139 • Preimplantation Genetic Diagnosis (PGD) 140 • Surrogates and Gestational Care 141 • ZIFT (Zygote Intrafallopian Transfer) 143 • Other Things to Consider When Choosing Infertility Treatment 144

8. Telling Friends and Family ..................................... 149

WELCOME TO LAND-MINE CITY!

Who to Tell and What to Say 151 • How to Cope with Insensitive Comments 153 • How to Cope with Social and Work Obligations 156

9. Affording Infertility ............................................ 160

EVEN MILLIONAIRES THINK THIS PART HURTS

The Ins and Outs of Health Insurance 162 • Insurance Checklist 167 • Shared-Risk or Money-Back-Guarantee Programs 168 • Other Ways to Save Money or Pay for IVF 174 • How to Handle Other Infertility Financial Nightmares 176 • Loss of Insurance Coverage 176 • Paying for Medication 177 • Time off from Work 178

10. Becoming Your Own Advocate .............................. 180

YOU GO, GIRL!

11. Understanding Your Cycle ................................... 185

INFERTILITY TREATMENT EXPLAINED FOR NON–ROCKET SCIENTISTS

Medications 186 • Protocols (IVF Only) 191 • Injections 193 • Side Effects 196 • Going in for Training 197

12. Beginning Your Infertility Treatment ..................... 200

IT'S EXCITING FOR ABOUT A DAY

Getting Going 200 • Creating a Care Package 204 • Living Through the Cycle 205 • Everything up to and Including the Day of Your HCG Trigger Injection 207 • Monitoring: How's My Cycle Progressing? 208 • Managing Stress 216 • IUI Patients: Everything from Insemination to Fertilization 219 • IVF Patients: Everything about Retrieval 220 • Embryo Quality, Day-3, Day-5, and Day-6 Blastocyst Transfers, and Assisted Hatching Explained 223 • IVF Patients and Embryo Transfer 228 • Frozen Embryo Transfers (FET) 230 • The Dreaded Two-Week Wait 233 • Your Pregnancy Test 235

13. Finding Out If Your Cycle Was Successful ............... 236

IS THIS THE MOST STRESSFUL TIME OF YOUR LIFE OR WHAT?

All About Betas and Home Pregnancy Tests 236 • You're Pregnant! 240 • Negative
Betas, Failed Cycles, and Miscarriage 242

14. Deciding When It's Time to Move On .................... 247

ENOUGH, ALREADY!

15. Making Your Infertility Work for You .................... 253

YES, INFERTILITY CAN BE A GOOD THING


*Appendix* ........................................................ 255

*Resources* ....................................................... 275

*Index* ........................................................... 281

# Foreword

As a reproductive endocrinologist and infertility specialist at the Center for Reproductive Medicine and Infertility, Weill Medical College of Cornell University, I have treated thousands of infertile couples, every one of whom could benefit from this comprehensive, emotionally honest, and insightful book.

Written by a patient whose expertise consists of her actual experience with infertility—and the many treatments she underwent—*The Infertility Survival Handbook* speaks in the honest, knowing and emotionally incisive voice so many of my patients have often searched in vain to find.

The author, Liz Swire Falker, was my patient for four years. In her quest to have a biological child during that time, Liz underwent numerous surgeries, procedures, treatments, and pregnancy losses. Her *Infertility Survival Handbook* may be the first authoritative book on infertility treatment from the point of view of one who has been there.

In the first section, Liz opens her heart and relives her own experiences. Her fearless and generous firsthand account will give infertile couples a good sense of what may be ahead for them as they try to conceive. Liz's depictions of her interactions with her husband, family, friends, and physicians during the course of her treatment will also give current patients a useful, and ultimately reassuring, guide.

Giving medical and nonmedical aspects of infertility treatment equal attention, Liz provides detailed discussions of all aspects of infertility treatment, from IUI and IVF, to unusual ways of financing treatment. And she does so in a manner that is practical and supportive, and that should help patients stay sane and focused during what can be a very difficult process.

As a physician in this field, I can assure you that the information in this book is accurate and updated. Just as important to the patients who look to these pages, Liz has an amazing ability to present highly technical information in a way that is accessible to general readers.

In addition to being a good source of medical information, *The Infertility Survival Handbook* provides what I know can be a welcome source of information and encouragement to couples dealing with infertility issues. Invariably, some are luckier than others. For those who do not successfully conceive, even after extensive treatment, the book offers advice, strategies, and outright wisdom to help survive their fury and grief.

Finally, couples who struggle with infertility and the challenges it presents can have a book they deserve and trust.

Pak H. Chung, M.D.
New York
August 2003

# Acknowledgments

There are so many people who have touched my life while I underwent infertility treatment and during the time I wrote this book. Mostly, I would like to thank my mother; without her support this book never would have been written. To my father, thank you for teaching and encouraging me to write.

To my agent, Bob Tabian, I am profoundly grateful that you understood exactly what this book is about and believed in it. To Sandi Gelles-Cole, thank you for all your insight and guidance getting the first draft of this book ready. And my many thanks to my editor, Susan Lehman, who helped a lawyer sound like a human being.

To the staff at The Center for Reproductive Medicine and Infertility, my sincere thanks for your friendship, patience, and support during four of the most emotionally demanding years of my life. To Lila, Marianne, Marcie, Vickie, Rosanna, and the entire IVF nursing and technical staff, thank you for taking such good care of me and being so supportive through my ups and downs; thanks for putting up with me! To Drs. Zev Rosenwaks, Steven Spandorfer, Orli Etingin, and all the superlative physicians, fellows, embryologists, and andrologists on staff, thank you for contributing your acumen and skill to my attempts to have a biological child and carry a pregnancy to term. To Barbara and Linda, thank you for helping me keep my head screwed on straight throughout this ordeal.

To Cari, my eternal thanks for holding my hand when Charlie couldn't. To Cathy, Donna, Leigh Ann, Lisanne, Lynn, Karen, Kathryn,

Sheila, Tara, and Vickee, thank you for always being there, listening to me, and guiding me with your wisdom and strength. You have all taught me more about friendship and sisterhood than you will ever know.

To the staff at the Rye (and Larchmont) Starbucks for my most delicious daily iced decaf venti skim extra mocha extra ice double cup mocha, and to Tom for always finding me a comfy chair near an outlet for my laptop.

To Dr. Pak H. Chung . . . there are no words to thank you for *all* that you have done to help me achieve my dream of being a mother. Thank you for your unending support, compassion, friendship, patience, and honesty. You are a *gifted* physician and healer, and I am profoundly grateful that you cared for me during such a difficult period of my life. You enriched my life and eased my suffering in ways you cannot comprehend. Thank you from the bottom of my heart.

To Charlie, my husband, soul mate, and father of my son, I could not ask for more in a partner. You bless me every day. Thank you for your willingness to take our infertility treatment to the outer limits of sanity and medical science. Because of your patience, acceptance, and understanding, I am more at peace as a human being and a mother. Thank you for helping me hold the door shut!

# Introduction

There isn't any getting around it: having trouble getting pregnant sucks. Watching your friends conceive almost the minute they start trying when you've been trying for what feels like forever (and may very well have been forever), hurts. Your friends with newborns talk about nursing, diaper rash, nannies, balancing work and baby, and sleepless nights. You sit mute and jealous. If you offer any advice, your friends look at you with that "you just don't understand because you don't have a baby" expression. Friends with babies can't go out with you and your husband. In fact, forget about seeing them, unless it's at Saturday afternoon Gymboree.

Your pregnant friends (who all seem to be on baby number two or three by now) complain about how fat they are, how much the baby is kicking, how insensitive their husbands are, and how awful it is to be pregnant—or worse—pregnant *again*. You want to scream! Why can't they shut up and realize how lucky they are? You would give your left arm and right leg to be pregnant.

I don't know about you, but members of my family have been the most difficult to deal with. We didn't tell our families when we first started trying to have a baby. Big mistake! My mother must have asked me when we would have a baby in *every* conversation we had. But the minute I finally confided and told her we were having problems conceiving, she shut up. I could have spared myself *so* much grief had I just said something earlier! How weird; now that I wanted to talk to her about it, I couldn't get her to stay on the subject for more than a millisecond. This is one of the many no-win aspects of baby-making land.

Family members aren't the only ones driving you crazy. I can't begin to count the number of friends and family members Charlie (my husband) and I stopped seeing because of our infertility. We can't relate to their lives, and they don't understand anything about the hell we've been living through. Sometimes you share your experience with a couple that admits that they, too, experienced infertility, or you find that one of your friends is particularly sensitive and can be supportive and comforting while her baby screams in the background. But most of my good friends seemed to get pregnant at the drop of their pants, and I just couldn't deal with it. What's it like to get pregnant the first month you try (or by *accident*) and be freaked out that you aren't ready to be a mother? I wish I knew.

I have one or two friends who had problems starting a family, but both these women had difficulty staying pregnant (something that I now appreciate, having had several miscarriages), but not getting pregnant. Both have been very supportive, and one of my oldest friends really "gets" what I am going through. But for the most part, I really don't have any friends who truly understand what the surgeries are for, or the shots, what the shots did to me emotionally (not to mention physically), or how emotionally draining (not to mention expensive) infertility treatment and adoption can be. I get support from the infertile women I have met over the Web or at my doctor's office. A couple of these women have become very dear friends. They always know what to say to boost my morale. You will find this is important when you're going through this stuff, because most of the time friends and family say the wrong thing—even those who mean well—and it hurts a lot.

Don't feel guilty if you find you are suddenly judging friends and family members by new standards. When you are infertile, there are two classes of people: those who understand how hard it is and those who don't. If you feel the need to stop communicating with insensitive or unsupportive people, do it! And don't feel guilty about it, either. Do what you have to in order to get through this time in your life. It's okay to be selfish right now.

Don't let guilt get in the way of anything, especially not your sex life! After trying to conceive for a few months, even those who know the art of the *Kama Sutra* find sex annoying, boring, and time-consuming. If you are still trying to conceive the old-fashioned way and find your marriage and sex life are straining under the stress, I have one suggestion for you: soft pornography. I can't tell you how many of my friends found this really helped them conceive. Don't be embarrassed; there is a huge market of adult videos for a reason (some are even made for women, with romance and seduction as part of the almost nonexistent plot). If you're past trying the adult video section, well, have faith, your sex life will come back (before the baby is born), but it takes a while. If you're living through surgeries and tests, don't expect to have the urge to jump your hubby's bones. If your husband doesn't get it, ask him how romantic he feels after a prostate exam! Eventually sex will be fun again, I promise. And when you start down the path of assisted reproductive technologies, there's one not-so-little bonus to look forward to. All the fertility meds you'll be taking might make you rather horny! Does it surprise you that drugs that cause major hormonal shifts (within hours of ingesting or injecting them) would also make you want to have all kinds of illicit sex? Well, get over it, so you can get your sex life back!

Lastly, don't feel guilty about the fact that the urge to have a baby consumes you. This is *normal* for *all of us*. Your day revolves around calculating where you are in your menstrual cycle, what your basal body temperature is, how much cervical fluid you have and what consistency it is, whether or not to use a third ovulation predictor kit that day, or—even more challenging—how many days you have to wait until you take a pregnancy test. If you're close to the end of the cycle, you run to the bathroom every five seconds to wipe and see if there is any blood. You give yourself toilet paper burn and cause more than a few raised eyebrows among your coworkers as you run to the bathroom for the twenty-seventh time that morning.

If you're further along the infertility path, you may be obsessing about what next procedure is scheduled to help diagnose your problem. And as you advance to what I consider "platinum" infertility status—you have now spent so much money treating your infertility that your credit card company has offered you a platinum card—you spend your days racing to the fertility clinic to get blood work and an ultrasound, and waiting for the inevitably tardy afternoon phone call from the nurse at your clinic with your dosage instruction for your evening injection. It feels like everything in your life hinges on that phone call. And if you've decided to adopt, your life revolves around a cell phone that is connected to an 800 number that only prospective birth mothers know (and may call at any time of the day or night) or waiting for the day's mail with your international adoption referral. You jump every time that cell phone rings and check your watch a thousand times to see if the mail might have been delivered. Obsession knows nothing compared to the angst of an infertile woman in wait. This is *all* normal.

Through all of this, the important thing to remember is that *you are not alone.* Countless women have and will ride the infertility roller coaster. They survived, and so will you. Some have even made it through and actually feel that their infertility was a gift. My infertility has changed my life in many profound ways. I have learned so much about myself and about patience, compassion, and love that, in retrospect, I might actually do it all over again. I would rather not stab myself three or four times a day with needles and/or feel powerless and at the mercy of a pregnant seventeen-year-old contemplating placing her baby for adoption. But Charlie and I have worked through so many issues in our marriage and are so much closer now; and it's because of our infertility.

My husband and I know how to talk and listen to each other and to be there for each other. Our infertility has taught us this. There's something about feeling all alone against the world (not to mention spending some hard time in marriage counseling discussing this stuff) to give you a new sense of commitment in your marriage. The only other person on this earth who knows the pain inside my heart is Charlie. I have learned how to share my grief with him in counseling, and he has learned how to comfort me. He has been there for me in the recovery room after surgery, in the bathroom in the middle of the night after surgery (throwing up from anesthesia), in bed late at night after embryo transfer when my fear of failing is the strongest, waiting for pregnancy test results and when I am mourning the loss of a child (through miscarriage or a failed adoption). I do not hide these feelings from him, and he shares most of his with me. Infertility brings out strong, almost primal emotions in each of us, and we have learned to let those emotions teach us about ourselves and each other, and make us stronger. It hasn't been easy to learn to share like this (I do think my husband is slightly more evolved than most men, but maybe I'm wrong), but it has helped us. And our son is benefiting from this. That's right, I have a baby!

Our son, David, is the most loved, most wanted, most cherished child on the planet (I think that all infertile couples feel this way). We battled entire armies of demons to have him. In addition to the sometimes overwhelming difficulties and frustrations we endured during our infertility treatment, David's adoption was fraught with challenges I didn't know how I would overcome (as you will learn, sometimes you just have to take it one step at a time or even one moment at a time). But once my baby was in my arms, I realized every second of my struggle and every stick of every needle was worth it. He is my miracle!

Having and raising children means more to me now than it would have if I had gotten pregnant on the first try. I worked really hard to have this family. My life changed enormously because I am infertile. I am more mature, more peaceful, more grounded in who I am and who I want to be because I am infertile. I am more committed to my long-term health and spiritual well-being than I was before this hell took over my life. I gave up my career to do IVF (being a litigator doesn't give one a lot of time for daily injections, blood tests, and ultrasounds, not to mention mood swings or extended absences from work for egg retrieval and embryo transfer), and in the process I found myself. I had no idea that I was so unhappy being a lawyer. Nor did I realize just how much I wanted to be a mother. "Babylust" doesn't even begin to cover it.

I realized that motherhood is one of my highest goals. It is a gazillion times more important to me than winning trials and being the best lawyer I can be. Much of my sense of self as a woman involves being a mother, breast-feeding, and cleaning up stinky poop (surprisingly, it doesn't bug me, and this is coming from someone with a *major* gag reflex), not in arguing for some company's right to fire its employee or breach a contract. Had I not struggled with infertility, I would've been horribly conflicted when it came time to juggle family responsibility and career. There is no question that my life will be forever different because I quit my career; financially, it will never be the same. I am a full-time mother, and to me that's as important as being a senior partner at the nation's most prestigious law firm. Heck, it's more important.

Despite the profound growth I've experienced as a result of having major infertility issues, I don't want you to believe for a minute that this has been easy for me. When I say that being infertile is hell, I mean *hell*. This has been the most physically grueling and emotionally draining experience of my life. It's been more than a year since I discontinued infertility treatment and had my last miscarriage, and I still wrestle with my weight (the infertility drugs), with our finances (this stuff is so expensive), and with my attitude (you'll discover that attitude is everything). Even when I'm rocking David to sleep at night, I continue to battle my fear and anger that I might never feel a baby grow inside my belly for nine (really ten) months. Those emotions resurface despite the fact that I know in my heart and my soul that David was meant to be my son, whether I gave birth to him or someone else did.

And what really irks me is that I have to face the same issues all over again if I want to add a sibling to our little family. Should we adopt again (how will we pay for it?), should I go back into treatment (will insurance cover it?), should we try an IVF surrogacy (where someone else carries our biological child)? Infertility does *not* go away. I have gotten pregnant, I've miscarried, I've survived failed adoptions, and I've endured experiences and emotions I never knew existed, and sometimes I feel like it will never end. This is the hell to which I refer and that I continue to endure. But this is the hell from which I emerged a stronger, more centered woman, and a mother.

I wrote this book because I don't believe infertility needs to be such a struggle. First of all, it doesn't have to be so lonely. Second, it seems to me that someone needs to share the secrets of assisted reproductive technologies (ART) like intrauterine insemination (IUI), in vitro fertilization (IVF), and adoption (not to mention a few other things). It's as if there's a secret handbook that you get only after you've done IVF a bazillion times and talked to a trillion birth mothers (like I have). There is a lot you learn from going through infertility treatment more than once, and a lot you learn once you've gone through one adoption (we've actually attempted more than one). My doctor's nurse teases me about how thick my medical chart is (I don't appreciate that, by the way), but I know a lot of the secrets of infertility-land from having a chart that thick. (It's almost as thick as Webster's Unabridged Dictionary; how depressing is that?) And my adoption caseworker laughs with me about the number of birth mothers I've spoken to and worked with toward an adoption (it's called gallows humor), but I'm now an "expert" when it comes to building a family. There is certainly a lot I would've done differently if I'd known what was ahead and what it all meant before I made expensive (both emotionally and financially) decisions.

I hope that I can give you the benefit of my experience so that you can make the best choices possible for you and your partner. I also hope this book becomes a resource for you, helps you to navigate the maze of infertility tests and treatments, and enables you to handle the various financial and marital stresses that accompany infertility treatment. I will explain what endometriosis and what PCOS are, and stuff like that (you need to understand what's wrong with you to know what decisions to make about treatment) and try to give you some advance warning about different tests and treatments. We'll talk about asking your doctor and nurse questions and being your own advocate for your medical care. And we'll talk about IUIs and IVF in detail and also discuss traditional adoption, embryo donation, donor eggs (and sperm), gestational surrogacy, and living child-free. I'll try to remind you—as often as possible—just how normal it is to feel as if you're losing your mind (not to mention your waistline). If you need more information about endometriosis, male-factor infertility, or anything else, please check out the Resources section at the back of the book.

Whether you get pregnant on your first IUI, your sixth IVF cycle, or one day decide to adopt or live without children, I hope you find something in this book that resonates for you and eases your grief. Yes, infertility sucks. But it won't suck forever, and it doesn't have to suck every day.

# Telling My Story

As I write, Charlie and I have been trying to conceive for more than seven years and recently adopted our son, David. Motherhood is awesome, but my journey toward motherhood and my continuing efforts to enlarge our family have been arduous, to say the least. It started the way it starts for many people, with arguments over when we would start our family. I really wanted to start a family early; our honeymoon would've been perfect (not to mention romantic). Charlie was a little bit reluctant to have kids. It took him a long time to come around and really get into the whole fatherhood gig. I am happy to say that being a dad suits him, and I think many of those men who seem reluctant ultimately turn into the best fathers on the planet (at least mine did). But getting here hasn't exactly been that romantic vision I had for my life.

About nine years ago, after fighting about it for a long time, Charlie finally agreed to start trying to have a baby. Almost immediately my menstrual cycles went crazy. My OB-GYN recommended that I start charting my basal body temperature (also known as BBT to those of us who use the Internet as a support resource) to see if I was ovulating. I ran to CVS and bought a digital basal thermometer, downloaded a BBT chart off the Web, and went to work each morning taking my temp. My temperatures were all over the place. There's supposed to be this neat little temperature rise after ovulation, but I seemed to have a BBT pattern more like a roller coaster (a preview of the hell to come, perhaps?). My OB-GYN appeared stumped (I now know that the pattern on my chart pretty much presented a no-brainer of a diagnosis, so the fact that she couldn't figure it out should have tipped me off that I needed a new OB-GYN), and referred me to a reproductive endocrinologist (RE). Had my doctor been more involved or just plain smarter—as I would soon discover—I could have tried a fairly quick and easy fix.

When I told Charlie that I needed to see a specialist, he got tense (that puts it mildly). He asked me to wait a little while before starting "all of that" and just "relax." God, I *hate* such patronizing comments! I complied. Then, after almost a year of trying to conceive our first child— my BBT was still all over the place, I was lobbying aggressively to see a specialist, and our marriage was getting extremely unfriendly—Charlie told me that he wasn't sure he could continue to try. He wasn't sure he wanted children! This was not what I wanted to hear (understatement of the *century*). You can probably imagine my reaction (not pretty).

Okay. I am going to stop here, because this stuff starts to get super personal, and our specific issues aren't necessarily relevant to your concerns. Suffice it to say that we went into marriage counseling, worked out this not-so-little-issue, and started trying to conceive again a couple of years later. If you're having problems in your relationship because of infertility, remember that most people do experience stress from this, and if you're open to it, marriage counseling or individual counseling can be a *big* help. By the way, the time we were in marriage counseling does not count as part of my many years in infertility hell. One other note about this period of time: the minute we stopped trying, I demonstrated my first normal BBT chart. Ironic, yes? Or perhaps it was just part of the greater plan (definitely part of the greater plan).

Just before we started trying again, I switched to a wonderful OD-GYN, Dr. M. (We'll call her Dr. Marvelous because I think that's what she is.) I had been a patient of Dr. Marvelous in the past and had left her care when she stopped accepting insurance (but I was now willing to spend money to see someone I trusted). She looked at the BBT charts, looked at me, and said quite matter-of-factly, "You weren't ovulating."

Like I said, kind of a no-brainer. We talked about trying Clomid, a fairly low-tech fertility drug, but since my cycles had been regular for a while, she suggested that we give it some time. She recommended that I stop charting and instead try using an ovulation predictor kit (Web shorthand: OPK). Considering how unromantic that digital thermometer was, I thought this an excellent suggestion. I ran out to CVS and bought my first OPK. We officially started trying again.

Months went by. I had perfectly normal cycles and would get a positive indicator on the OPK and my period fourteen days later. Sometimes I felt like something might have happened (and drive Charlie crazy with my obsessive excitement), but then my period would be right on time. I was disappointed and frustrated and then perplexed. I was doing everything right, so what was wrong? I went back to Dr. Marvelous. She said that everything seemed normal, and we should give it a few more months and then try Clomid. But, she warned me, before I could take Clomid, I would have to have a diagnostic procedure to make sure my fallopian tubes are open (no point giving me a drug to help me ovulate if my tubes are blocked and there is nowhere for the egg to go to meet the sperm), and the procedure can be unpleasant (and when a doctor says "unpleasant," whoa girl! Watch out!). The procedure is called a hysterosalpingogram (HSG for short), and I discuss it in detail in chapter 4.

Between the thought of an unpleasant test and general denial that I might have a serious fertility problem (we've all been there, yes?), Charlie and I kept trying for quite a bit longer. I even started charting my BBT again with the support of some friends on a fertility-oriented Web site. No matter how many months passed, I was lulled into the sense that it was okay it was taking so long because there was "always next month." Denial doesn't help those of us trying to have a baby without success. It is one thing not to want to admit you're having problems (who wants to acknowledge that?), but letting *more* time go by when there is a serious problem isn't a good idea.

I have so many friends who waited until their mid to late thirties before trying to conceive. First months, then years went by; when they finally found out something was wrong and sought treatment for male-factor infertility or blocked fallopian tubes, they also had to contend with ovaries that were more interested in retiring than in producing eggs or other issues connected to what doctors commonly—and horrendously—call "advanced maternal age." These women regretted waiting a day (let alone the months or years they waited) to get treatment. Don't let this be you! If you are over thirty-five, don't wait. If you aren't pregnant, run—do not walk—to your OB-GYN. Here's one rule of thumb from my beloved OB-GYN: If you aren't pregnant in six months, see your doctor. The one-year rule is just *wrong*. My own denial is something I regret.

Finally, after a lovely vacation with Charlie during peak ovulation time, my period was late and my temperature was elevated for sixteen days past ovulation. My books and on-line support group told me this was a sign I was pregnant. But my home pregnancy tests (HPTs) were all negative. I called Dr. Marvelous. She told me to give it a few more days, assume I was pregnant, and come in for a pregnancy test in about a week. Two more days went by with elevated temps (when I hit what they say is the positive pregnancy BBT mark, eighteen elevated temps past ovulation) and no period, but still no positive HPT. I was so excited, and then—well, you know that familiar little sensation in the middle of your lower abdomen—*cramps!* I scrambled to the bathroom (in the middle of an important meeting, of course) and discovered that I had my period. I managed not to cry until I got home that night, and then I wept in Charlie's arms for about an hour. I was devastated.

My cramps were horrible, and the bleeding was nasty and didn't stop when it should have. Finally my period ended, and then just as quickly began again. I started bleeding every two weeks. I called Dr. Marvelous, who quickly discovered a cyst on my ovary. She sent me for an ultrasound, which revealed something that I had long feared; I probably had endometriosis (known to those with the dreaded disease as "endo"). •

My mother's whole family has endo. I am an only child because of endo. I was deeply, *deeply* afraid of endometriosis. Dr. Marvelous scheduled me for a laparoscopy (I tell you about what this surgical procedure is in chapter 4), which confirmed that I have severe endo. One of my fallopian tubes appeared permanently scarred shut with adhesions, my uterine cavity was a mass of fibroids and polyps (Dr. Marvelous wasn't surprised I hadn't gotten pregnant or hadn't been able to stay pregnant with all that stuff in there), there were adhesions on my bowel, bladder, everywhere. How could I not have felt this? (I've always had bad cramps, you get used to it, you know?) Dr. Marvelous referred me to a fertility clinic.

I am very lucky to live near one of the world's best fertility clinics. When Dr. Marvelous referred me to the Center for Reproductive Medicine and Infertility at Cornell Medical College (CRMI), she wasn't fooling around. The men and women at CRMI are—in my acknowledged biased opinion (but the unbiased agree with me as well)—some of the best fertility docs in the world. That is not to say that CRMI hasn't made mistakes and that there aren't other amazing clinics and independent REs out there; I have interviewed several of them for this book and for second opinions. But after you hear everything I've gone through to have a baby, I think you will see why I think CRMI, and my personal RE in particular, are so worth my prejudice. There are a lot of charlatans and idiots out there in baby-making land, and finding the best possible fertility doctor you can is extremely important (I devote some time to discussing this in chapter 3); I was lucky to wind up at CRMI right from the beginning.

Amazingly enough, I only had to wait five weeks to get an appointment with one of the female REs on staff at CRMI. (As you may discover, a six-month wait or longer is common at many of the big fertility centers.) Charlie and I met with Dr. I (hereinafter known as Dr. Motormouth as she spoke more quickly than anyone I've ever met before). Immediately Charlie said that he couldn't understand a word she said and didn't care for her bedside manner (she wasn't exactly warm); but she was going to be my physician, so he didn't think his opinion should matter that much. In retrospect, I should have followed his gut instinct and met with someone else at the clinic. I was about to learn something about ignoring the personal side of a doctor.

Dr. Motormouth told me in vitro fertilization (IVF) offered me the best chance of conception. Charlie and I weren't ready, psychologically, for IVF and asked if we could we start with something less medically invasive. IVF also is expensive, and we weren't financially prepared for it. But I think the biggest issue for me was that I saw IVF as a technology of last resort, something I would learn later on is wrong, wrong, wrong. IVF is, and should be, considered a first-line treatment for many couples (there's more on this in chapter 7). I wasn't ready to face the depth and degree of my own infertility.

Dr. Motormouth agreed to start with ovulation induction and intra-uterine inseminations (IUIs). She suggested one more diagnostic procedure (the HSG that Dr. Marvelous had warned me was unpleasant), and despite a lot of complaining (I had barely just recovered from my laparoscopy), I agreed. I scheduled the HSG and mentally prepared myself for the test. I bribed myself with thoughts of a shortened workday, a fabulous postprocedure dinner and, if needed, lots of good painkillers.

Despite extraordinary pain, the HSG was a success. Dr. Motormouth managed to open the fallopian tube that Dr. Marvelous thought was permanently scarred shut. That HSG was worth suffering through to have two fully functioning fallopian tubes. Next stop, fertility drugs and IUIs.

I was tremendously excited. I felt like I had my first real chance to conceive a baby. As I started the fertility medication and daily routine of ultrasounds and phone calls with the clinic, I began to notice how stressful and time-consuming my job as a litigator was. Suddenly making my doctor's appointment was more important than meeting court-scheduled deadlines. My bosses' complaints about late-morning arrivals (morning ultrasound and blood draws) or not staying late enough at night (nightly injections) seemed petty and insignificant. I had worked very hard for my career, but I also had worked very hard to get to a point physically where I could have a child. My desire to be a mother grew stronger with each injection. So did the tension and resentment I felt toward my employers. Something would have to give.

Charlie and I started talking about my near-stratospheric stress levels. I had been unhappy with my current job for a long time and had wanted to find a new one. The time demands now placed on me because of the infertility treatment made interviewing impossible, and staying at my current position was almost unfathomable. But we couldn't afford for me not to work; I was the primary wage earner in our family. Charlie was extremely supportive. We agreed that I would quit my job and start working as a temporary or contract attorney. The money would be less, but I would have more flexibility. I also decided to take some time off before I started work again. Just before I left my job, my first IUI cycle failed. I was horribly disappointed but also felt that the stress connected with the job change probably prevented me from getting pregnant, as studies consistently show that high stress levels reduce the success rates for ART (for more on stress management, see chapter 12). I was sure I'd get pregnant after I quit my job. But three IUIs later, I wasn't pregnant and Dr. Motormouth was leaving my clinic.

Charlie and I started interviewing other doctors in New York City. Other clinics were unbelievably aggressive in trying to get our business (I don't believe interviewing an RE should feel like you're shopping for a used car), or had facilities that were so filthy I was afraid to walk barefoot on the exam room floor (we'll talk about selecting a doctor in chapter 3). We decided to switch to Dr. Pak H. Chung, another physician at CRMI.

At our first meeting, Dr. Chung really impressed us. He was compassionate and thoughtful and had spent a lot of time reviewing my medical history. He listened, answered questions, and was sympathetic and optimistic, yet realistic. For the first time during my infertility treatment, I felt I had met a physician who truly cared about me and wanted me to get pregnant. On the way home from our first visit with Dr. Chung, I cried. I felt recognized and understood.

Dr. Chung told me I needed more surgery before continuing treatment. He also encouraged us to move on to IVF. I agreed to surgery, a hysteroscopy (see chapter 4) to remove uterine polyps, but expressed my desire to try one or two more IUIs before moving on to IVF. Dr. Chung understood that I still was not ready to make the emotional leap to IVF and felt that it was reasonable to do one or two more inseminations.

I did one natural cycle IUI (no fertility drugs) that same month, which was unsuccessful. The following month I went ahead with the hysteroscopy, and two months after that, I did one last IUI with fertility meds.

Again, I failed to get pregnant. Dr. Chung told us that CRMI believes that if a patient doesn't get pregnant after three or four tries with IUI or IVF, it's time to move on. I had now had four failed IUIs; it was time for IVF. It had been eight months and two surgical procedures since I became an infertility patient and started using high-tech help, and I had been trying to have a baby for well over three years. I welcomed IVF and the new hope it offered for a baby.

I was supposed to have gone back to work by this point, but it never happened. I was offered some great temporary gigs, but I couldn't do it. The procedures, the medication, and the surgeries were too much. I could barely cope with the infertility treatment and couldn't imagine how I would fit work into an IVF schedule. I even turned down one job that I would have killed for a couple of years earlier. Charlie was supportive, but we were both concerned about our finances. It was tough enough to be going through infertility, but trying to pay for it without my income was frightening. My parents and my in-laws offered to help. As a temporary, stopgap measure, their help enabled us to continue infertility treatment, but it didn't begin to solve long-term issues presented by my loss of income. We were going to have to make some hard choices.

I realized it was time I made some decisions about how much I was willing to put myself through to have a baby grow inside my belly. Dr. Chung was very optimistic about our chances of having a baby with IVF. I considered his optimism, Charlie's confidence (a confidence I was not quite able to share all of the time), and decided to go for it. I would do everything humanly and medically possible to get pregnant, deliver a child into this world, and breast-feed. We would tighten our belts and pray that insurance would cover most of the expenses (you need to do more than pray when it comes to insurance, a fact I discuss in chapter 9).

Dr. Chung explained that the next step was to have Charlie get a more specialized semen analysis, a Kruger analysis. Charlie had had many semen analyses done in the past, and everything seemed okay. None of the prior tests, however, looked at the shape of his sperm as carefully as this test would. There would be no point in doing IVF with Charlie's sperm unless we knew his sperm could do the job. The Kruger analysis would tell us whether Charlie's sperm could fertilize my eggs, or whether they would need help from a technique known as ICSI (intracytoplasmic sperm injection, which is discussed in chapter 6).

Now let's take a moment and talk about the acronyms and huge words infertility docs toss around. It is hard to absorb all these shorthand references for high-tech procedures, but knowing what they mean and how to use them really helps. If patients and doctors had to use the polysyllabic, tongue-twisting names for all this stuff, they'd spend all their time with you just trying to get one sentence out. It's also a badge of honor (okay, it's not like winning the Pulitzer or anything, but it makes you feel like an insider) when you can use these words and abbreviations correctly in a sentence. Your doctor will be impressed, and you will feel empowered (my God, she has a *brain!*). I bet you can't use ICSI, HSG, IVF, and Kruger all in one sentence, correctly. I can, and it's something I take pride in. How twisted is that? I'll demonstrate for you in a moment.

Charlie went ahead with the Kruger analysis, and I went over instructions for my first IVF cycle with one of the IVF nurses. I'm a real baby when it comes to needles. I *hate* them. Nothing could've prepared me for the number of injections I would need for IVF or the size of the needle that someone (*Charlie?*) would have to stab into my behind *every day*. I was facing up to three injections a day, two in my lower abdomen (yes, that's right, my *lower abdomen*) and one in my derriere with a shockingly long needle. I was not a happy fertility camper.

While we waited for the IVF cycle to start, we got the results of Charlie's Kruger analysis. He had 0 percent morphology, or zero normal-shaped sperm. Apparently, sperm morphology (shape, which is what this test analyzes) is extremely important for fertilization. Funky-shaped sperm don't usually get the job done (although they can do it sometimes), and Charlie seemed to have an awful lot of funky-shaped sperm. The IVF nurse who gave me the results said we needed to talk to Dr. Chung about using donor sperm. Charlie and I both flipped out. After all the time we'd spent trying to deal with my fertility problems, we needed donor sperm? I was terribly confused. Charlie was devastated and angry. Neither one of us could understand why this hadn't been discovered earlier.

Dr. Chung called that night and explained that the IVF nurse I had spoken to was *wrong!* We didn't need donor sperm. It is possible to get pregnant (even the old-fashioned way) with severe morphology problems, but it's usually *much* more difficult—and sometimes it's impossible. To ensure that we achieved fertilization during IVF, we'd need to use a technique where they inject the sperm into the egg (called ICSI, pronounced IXSEE). Dr. Chung apologized profusely for the nurse's mistake and told us that he would personally see to it that every nurse on staff understood that 0 percent morphology meant only that ICSI was needed to achieve fertilization during IVF.

Dr. Chung also explained that the problems with Charlie's sperm's shape might explain why the IUI cycles had failed. Dr. Chung was very optimistic about ICSI and my prognosis. So now, after the painful laparoscopy and HSG, my endo diagnosis and four failed IUIs, the Kruger suggested that maybe our fertility problems weren't *my* problem after all! We probably just needed IVF and ICSI all along. (See, I told you I could do it, and I even threw in a few other big words to impress you!)

As an aside, I've got to say that if you're going to make a mistake in baby-making land when telling someone the results of a fertility test, male-factor (sperm) infertility isn't the best place to screw up. Women seem to be better able to take reproductive diagnoses (even horrible ones) in stride. Telling a man he can't impregnate his wife is about as low as it gets for a guy (see chapter 6 for more info on helping the infertile guy cope). And if you've already been doing infertility treatment for a while when you find out about a missed diagnosis, well, you're not just going to be freaked but more than a little frustrated! (I still don't understand why CRMI didn't do the Kruger earlier in our treatment.)

Once we recovered from the Kruger result fiasco, it was time to get going with our first IVF cycle. I've devoted an entire chapter to describing what IUI and IVF cycles feel like, but let me tell you right here, it was a shocker. No matter who you are or what your diagnosis is, IVF is incredibly challenging, physically and emotionally. Any woman who doesn't find IVF difficult should give Wonder Woman a run for her money.

My first IVF cycle failed, and I was devastated. Dr. Chung convinced us to try again. I took a few months off and spent the summer exercising and dieting to get rid of IVF-related weight gain (man, does that part *suck*). I also started going for acupuncture. I was surprised at how relaxing it was, and my second cycle seemed to go better. My estrogen level was lower (we talk about why this might be important in chapter 12), and while I produced fewer eggs than before, they were healthier this time, and we had better fertilization results. I believe the acupuncture had a lot to do with this; but don't ask a doctor to agree, because most of them think it's hooey. During the dreaded two-week wait at the end of the cycle, I started to feel something I hadn't experienced before (since that late period after my vacation). I was convinced I was pregnant. But the pregnancy test was negative.

As you may know (and will certainly learn soon enough) the second half of your menstrual cycle (or IUI/IVF cycle) is called the luteal phase (if you're a super medical geek like me and want the specifics on why it's called the *luteal* phase, read chapter 5). During the luteal phase of an IVF cycle, you are waiting to find out if you are pregnant; your doctor has transferred embryos to your uterus, and you are waiting to find out if they have implanted. This brings us to one of my personal IVF pet peeves: the common misconception that putting embryos into the uterus causes them to implant. It drives me crazy when people say that their doctor "implanted" four embryos. Embryos actually do the whole implantation thing by *themselves*. They do it by growing these tentacle-like extensions that reach into your uterine muscle to create an anchor for the embryo as it grows. These tentacle-like things also help the embryo gain access to your blood supply so that it can get nourishment before it has an umbilical cord and placenta to sustain it. And yes, this is important to understand; I'm not just trying to bore you. CRMI—being the very thorough and needle-loving folks that they are—can't just let you rest during your luteal phase. CRMI requires its patients to have two blood tests during this time (starting one week after embryo transfer), which analyze estrogen and progesterone levels. I personally think Dr. Chung subjected me to luteal blood work just to torture me. As if I needed more needles at a time in my IVF cycle when my stress level is at its peak.

These blood tests help determine whether they need to make adjust-ments in the medications you're taking and give an early peek to see if maybe, just maybe, you have an embryo burrowing in for a nice long nine- (okay, ten-) month stay. A third and final test when your period is due looks at pregnancy hormones, your beta HCG level (more medical lingo to learn), to see if that embryo has implanted and if you're pregnant.

When I spoke to Dr. Chung after getting my negative pregnancy test results, we talked about my luteal blood tests. Dr. Chung was able to see that an embryo had begun to implant, but that something may have dislodged it from my uterine wall. Dr. Chung wanted me to go see another doctor (Dr. Orli Etingin, vice chairman of Internal Medicine and a hematologist at New York Presbyterian Hospital—Cornell Medical Center) to see if I had an immune issue that was making it more difficult for an embryo to attach to my uterine wall or for it to grow once it is attached. (I talk in detail about this in chapters 4 and 5). Once again, in the middle of treatment, we were taking a detour into diagnostic stuff. I felt like we were taking two steps backward for every step forward.

Sure enough, after some more blood tests (more needles!) with Dr. Etingin, I found out that, due to a mutation of the MTHFR gene (be grateful I am using its initials, talk about polysyllabic, tongue-twisting hell!), I have a blood–clotting disorder. This disorder probably causes me to develop microscopic blood clots wherever the embryo's "tentacles" are trying to burrow into my uterine wall. These blood clots either cut off the blood supply to the embryo so that it can't grow or effectively dislodge the embryo from the uterine wall. There is also a nonreproductive medical disorder (called hyperhomocysteinenemia, sorry no shorthand for this one) caused by the gene mutation that causes heart disease and puts me at high risk for other medical problems, including having a baby with a neural tube defect. I am amazed that my infertility might have saved me from dying of heart disease! Fortunately, this blood–clotting disorder can be treated with baby aspirin, vitamin supplements, and injectible heparin, a prescription blood thinner (see chapter 5) to help me stay pregnant. My new IVF treatment protocol would require me to self-administer heparin once a day starting at the beginning of my IVF cycle and then increase to two injections per day after embryo transfer. I would have to continue this protocol until six weeks after the baby was born.

For once, I didn't care about more needles. (Did I mention what a needle-phobe I am?) I was just happy to have another explanation for my IVF failure. It's one of the twisted facts of the infertile woman's life; you're thrilled to have something wrong with you as long as it explains why you aren't getting pregnant! Dr. Chung was pleased to discover the MTHFR problem and now was even more optimistic about my prognosis. It turns out that the MTHFR issue may have been the biggest factor in our IUI and IVF failure, even with sperm issues and endo.

As we discussed starting my third IVF cycle, Dr. Chung and I realized that I was again experiencing quite a few endometriosis symptoms (now that I knew what they were). On top of the endo symptoms, he'd noticed during an ultrasound in my second IVF cycle that I again had uterine polyps and another ovarian cyst. After some noninvasive diagnostic tests (ultrasounds and the much more pleasant-to-live-through saline HSG, see chapter 4 for more detail), he decided I needed another laparoscopy. This was not good news. The first laparoscopy had taken weeks to recover from. It had been brutal. But the best time to get pregnant when you have endometriosis is the first six months to one year following a laparoscopy. I scheduled my second laparoscopy exactly one year and one week after my first one.

This time, the surgery wasn't too bad. I was up and moving around within a week, and I was glad I had gone through with it. Dr. Chung cleaned out all the adhesions and cysts from the endo, and my body was all ready for baby-making. While I was recovering from the surgery, I did some reading on the immune issues connected to endo (see the Resources section at the back of the book if you're interested in doing some additional reading) and the use of diet to help control the disease. I decided that it was a good time to make some dietary changes. I didn't want another laparoscopy. If I could keep the endo under control with diet, why not try?

So, about three months before the beginning of my third IVF cycle, I gave up dairy foods, food additives, colors and preservatives, alcohol, refined sugar, and stopped eating processed foods or anything containing partially hydrogenated oils. I started eating organic. I added vitamin supplements and started taking acidophilus and food enzymes. I felt better and even lost some weight. It is a hard diet to follow when you like cold cuts and cured meat as much I do (when I'm pregnant, I crave corned beef and pastrami sandwiches and often eat them for breakfast and lunch!), and in the long run I had to start eating dairy products again because I needed the calcium. But for the most part, I have kept to this diet, and though I can't be sure, I think it has slowed the progression of my endo. It has been almost three years since that last laparoscopy. The first two were a year apart, so this seems like progress to me!

My third IVF cycle was more emotionally difficult than the first two. What if the heparin didn't work, what if there was still something wrong with me, what if, what if, what if? After four IUIs and two IVFs, I couldn't face more failure. The cycle went well, however, and I wound up with extra embryos to freeze after transfer (a first for me).

And much to my own shock, I got pregnant. My first positive pregnancy test! Charlie and I were thrilled, ecstatic, overjoyed! My parents were thrilled! My in-laws were thrilled! Everyone was thrilled. This is what we had all been waiting for. It had all been worth it. I was going to have a baby!

But then my beta HCG level didn't rise normally. My HCG (this is the pregnancy hormone) level was initially low and was just barely doubling (it was supposed to at least double every forty-eight hours). I started living from blood test to blood test; my life seemed to move in forty-eight-hour increments. Finally, after almost a week, my beta quadrupled between tests. Dr. Chung called and congratulated us. He was happy and relieved. It seemed to be progressing into a healthy, normal pregnancy. It was Christmas, and he told me to enjoy the holidays and relax.

I was scheduled for an ultrasound and another pregnancy test the following week. I knew immediately when I saw the ultrasound screen that something was wrong. The doctor couldn't find a pregnancy sac, and there was a blood clot in my uterine cavity. I was numb. The doctor explained that it might just be too early to see a sac and that the morning's blood test would reveal more about the health of the pregnancy.

That night one of the nurses at CRMI called with the results of my blood test, and it wasn't good. My beta had barely doubled in a week. They asked me to repeat the blood work a week later. While waiting for the next test, I moved into automatic. I didn't feel anything, I just moved from one room to another, from one scene in my life to another. Motherhood seemed to be something that happened to other people.

After the next round of blood work, Dr. Chung was not optimistic about the pregnancy. Again, my beta HCG level had barely doubled in a week. It was barely 1,200 when it should have been over 15,000. At Dr. Chung's recommendation, I scheduled a D & C (a surgery to remove the pregnancy tissue) the following Monday. I started bleeding that Saturday afternoon, and my first pregnancy officially ended. I called Dr. Chung, and he told me to come in for the D & C on Monday; he wanted to make sure he removed all the pregnancy tissue.

I was miserable. Somewhere deep down inside me, I felt like I was dying. I was never going to be the same. Everything seemed a hurtful reminder of what I had lost. I had lost a child, I had lost my belief in my own reproductive abilities—in my ability to be a woman—and I had lost a sense of who I was as a human being. I wasn't a lawyer, I wasn't a mother, and I could barely function as a wife. What was I doing to myself?

I had an ultrasound the morning of my D & C, and Dr. Chung saw a small sac. I asked for a picture as a memento and to help me remember that it had been real. The picture helped me remember my "success." It became a talisman, a reminder of the fertility I didn't believe in.

After the D & C, we tried a frozen embryo cycle, but it didn't work. The drugs for the FET (another acronym, this one is for frozen embryo transfer, see chapter 12 for more info) cycle were far more brutal than for a fresh IVF cycle. As if it wasn't difficult enough managing the hormonal component of the FET and my fear of failure, I also developed monstrous hives wherever I injected the heparin. Dr. Etingin said I was one of the few people who are allergic to heparin. Why am I always the one with the weird or unusual diagnosis?

When the cycle failed, I was exhausted and horribly depressed. With my confidence shattered and my body a mess (from the miscarriage and the drugs from the frozen cycle), I had to decide whether to try again. Dr. Chung didn't have any easy answers. He did more tests and found that my uterine lining wasn't developing normally. We could increase the dosage of my progesterone injection just to be safe, but there was no way of knowing if it would make a difference. I was tired of not having answers. I decided to get some second opinions.

Getting second opinions turned out to be one of the best decisions I made in this entire process. First of all, I was shocked to learn how little some doctors know about fairly basic infertility issues. One of the doctors I spoke to didn't know what the MTHFR gene was! The doctors I sought opinions from were unanimous; CRMI was doing a great job for me. One doctor told me he would love my business, but he didn't think he could do as good a job for me as Dr. Chung was. If ever I had doubted my doctors, I didn't now. I returned to Dr. Chung, CRMI, and considerations of a new cycle with a fresh appreciation for what they had done for us.

After much soul searching, Charlie and I agreed to try another IVF cycle. I had some extra pathology testing done on the pregnancy tissue from my miscarriage and discussed trying some additional experimental therapies with Drs. Chung and Etingin. We decided to go ahead with the IVF cycle with the same protocol I had used before, but using a different injectable anticoagulant (Lovenox) because of the heparin allergy. I had gotten pregnant the first time I was treated for the MTHFR problem; there was nothing to indicate why I lost the pregnancy and nothing to indicate that we needed to make any substantive changes to warrant changing the IVF protocol. FET cycles commonly fail (we'll talk more about this in chapter 12, but generally speaking, frozen embryo transfers have much lower success rates than "fresh" IVF cycles do), and I was told that I shouldn't consider this indicative of my long-term prognosis. My prognosis was better than it had been a few months before because I had achieved a pregnancy.

I was skeptical and scared but wanted to try again. I was tired of asking, "What's wrong with me?" I was tired of being depressed and angry. I was tired of feeling barren. I wanted to prove to everyone that I could do this. But I was terrified that I would fail again.

My fourth IVF cycle was slightly more tolerable than my other three and far easier to deal with physically than the FET cycle had been (it was almost a relief to do a fresh IVF cycle). Mostly I had to deal with my own stupid issues: I was almost embarrassed to have been trying for so long, to have done so many fertility treatments. I saw a woman in the waiting room that I recognized from my IUI days; she was holding a small baby. Was it possible? Had I really been there long enough that she was back trying for number two? I saw a woman that I recognized from past IVF cycles. Had she failed, too, or miscarried? Did she recognize me? Did she know—as I did—how many months it had been since we had last been in the waiting room together? Where could I hide so she wouldn't see me and know what a failure I was?

The nurses at CRMI were all like sisters at this point. I had been a patient for so long I felt like they knew when I was getting my period before I did. I had even become very close friends with one nurse, Lila (one of the better things to come out of my infertility). The women who drew blood all knew me, and I had even established a relationship with one tech who was especially good at finding blood in my uncooperative arm. I had reached the point where I would only let two or three people touch me when it was time to draw blood. And I was ashamed. Ashamed that this was so difficult for me, that I couldn't handle it better and be an easier patient to deal with. Ashamed that they all knew me so well, ashamed that they pitied me, and ashamed of my inability to get pregnant. I felt stupid for coming back again and again for more humiliation. I felt like they looked at me and silently wondered why I didn't just give up. Didn't I know how futile this was?

I had definitely turned into a high-maintenance patient. But then again, after all those IUI and IVF cycles and four surgeries all within eighteen months, not to mention all the money I had paid CRMI (I still can't believe we managed to afford this), I felt I had earned a little extra attention. And for the most part, CRMI and its staff had been unbelievably caring and generous with me. They didn't treat me like the freak I feared I was (and frequently still do, even with lots of therapy). They treated me with respect and understanding. They knew this was my fourth IVF cycle; they knew what I was dealing with on a day-by-day basis, and despite my shame, fear, and frustration, they told me I was brave and strong and would be a wonderful mother.

And so my favorite tech drew my blood quickly and easily, and the nurses were extra careful to be supportive on the phone with my instructions, and Dr. Chung made an extra effort to do my ultrasounds every morning and check up on me when he had time. Without this extra attention, I wouldn't have been able to finish the cycle. My fourth IVF cycle was the most difficult of them all.

But the payoff was tremendous. I got pregnant again! And this time, when CRMI called with my pregnancy test results, my hormone levels were high. I was possibly carrying twins! I didn't even have to go in for more blood work for a week (unlike the previous pregnancy where I had to go in every forty-eight hours).

I was much more emotionally unstable than I had been during the last pregnancy. Part of this was fear, and part of it—unquestionably—was hormones. After a few days, I started to feel carsick all the time and then my breasts started to hurt. I started to have all the symptoms I read about in the books. Everything felt different from the last pregnancy and all the times I'd thought I was pregnant. I thought this must be the way a healthy pregnancy felt. My next round of blood work was fine. Everything was perfectly normal. *Finally!* I was pregnant, and it was okay to relax. We started looking at minivans (for fun), and I started reading baby books and pregnancy books. My first ultrasound was coming up, and we were so excited to see a heartbeat, or even two. Even Dr. Chung seemed excited!

The morning of my ultrasound I had a bad feeling. The bad feeling got worse as we got closer to the hospital. The ultrasound confirmed what I knew. Dr. Chung saw a sac, a yolk sac and a fetal pole (a baby), but no heartbeat (so much for twins). Charlie and I were devastated.

I cried from pain, anger, and confusion. I couldn't believe this was happening to me. Charlie looked shell-shocked. He wanted to cry (and may well have when I wasn't around) but held back—I think—so he wouldn't upset me further. The D & C was hell. I had to wait days to get a spot on Dr. Chung's OR schedule, and then the anesthesia made me violently ill. The pathology came back entirely normal, and as with my first miscarriage, the baby is presumed to have been a genetically normal little girl.

The following weeks were horrid. I moved as if under water. It was hard to breathe. I could barely function. For the first time in my life I seriously thought about how important having a biological child was. Was going through IVF and all that it entailed worth seeing Charlie's eyes or my smile in our baby? Why did pregnancy and childbirth seem so important? I started thinking that I might be happier if I gave up my dreams of pregnancy and instead adopted my children. But I wasn't ready to give up yet.

I obtained a consult from Carolyn Coulam, M.D., a leading reproductive immunologist. Together with her advice and Drs. Etingin and Chung, I decided to try an additional immune therapy, something called IVIG (discussed in chapter 5). We seemed to be moving into less and less medically tested territory. I was now heading into experimental therapies, and I was only willing to go so far with something that wasn't *proven* to work. This would be my last IVF cycle; if it failed, we would adopt. Dr. Chung agreed that if I didn't stay pregnant from the next cycle (assuming I even got pregnant) that he didn't hold out much hope for me to successfully carry a baby to term. He was honest and said that even if I hadn't decided to make it my last cycle, he was going to cut me off (no more IVF for this woman, at least not at CRMI). I felt much more peaceful having a finite ending point for treatment.

I started the IVIG therapy at the beginning of my next IVF cycle. It made me very sick, but if it meant that I might be able to carry a pregnancy to term, it was worth trying once. That cycle was canceled due to complications from ovarian hyperstimulation syndrome (OHSS), a dangerous and even life-threatening complication that can occur with IVF (see chapter 12 for more information). Feeling that I hadn't had a fair shot at trying the IVIG (I never even made it to egg retrieval), we decided to try it again.

I started my last IVF cycle—my sixth attempt, not including the FET. I was running on empty. I could barely function, and the thought of facing another loss was overwhelming. Now that I really knew what it felt like to be pregnant, Dr. Etingin and I determined that I probably had been pregnant at least twice on my own (I think it's really more like three times) and then three times with IVF. I couldn't take much more.

I completed my last cycle without complications and with a good number of healthy embryos. My pregnancy test was positive but very low; when it was repeated, it dropped. Clearly this was another nonviable pregnancy. I started bleeding a week later. That was—I believe—miscarriage number seven. But who's counting? We moved forward with our adoption plan.

Adoption was exciting and joy-filled at first. Within weeks of starting the process with our agency (The Gladney Center for Adoption; see the Resources section for information on this and other agencies) we had a birth mother who wanted us to parent her child. I was overwhelmed with joy and felt this was a sign that I was meant to adopt all along.

I still feel that way, but it turns out adoption was just as challenging as infertility treatment. Our first birth mother, "Diane*," decided to parent two hours before we were to receive placement (where the baby is given to you to take home). Diane called us back a few weeks later and asked us to parent, again. We agreed, and then Diane decided to parent, again. I worked on this book in the following months while we tried to find another birth mother. The day I finished the manuscript for this book, we matched (agreed to work exclusively) with another birth mother, "Heather.*"

---

*First names have been changed to protect individual's privacy.

It had now been six months since Diane had initially chosen to parent. I felt good about moving forward with another birth mother. Three days after matching with Heather, the agency called to tell us that Diane's son (now almost six months old) was legally available for adoption, and Diane still wanted us to parent him. We were on a plane a week later! As Diane has since told me, pictures from the day I held my son for the first time show a radiant, content woman. She's right! My son, David, is the light of my life and was worth waiting for and going through hell for. He was meant to be my son, and boy, did he try hard to get to us. I have no doubt that his soul always intended to be our child. When I couldn't maintain a pregnancy, David picked a very special woman to give him life and bring him home to us.

Never to do things the easy way, we continued to work with Heather on adopting her child as well. Heather gave birth a few months ago, and we had the immense pleasure and sadness of parenting her little boy for a few days. Ultimately, Heather chose to parent him. It was one of the hardest things (multiple miscarriages and David's initial failed adoption included) I've ever done, returning a child to his birth mother after I had nursed and loved him. Even so, I'm more at peace than I ever was during my infertility treatment.

While I'm thrilled to be a mother and even had the unique experience of inducing lactation and breast-feeding our adopted child (I induced lactation and pumped [and froze] breast milk for months for David and then relactated for the little boy we named Theo, and successfully breast-fed him for three days), I will never entirely heal from my miscarriages. My friends who've suffered multiple miscarriages tell me they feel the same way (for once I'm normal). These losses will stay with me forever, although time and distance have made them easier to bear. But I've got to be honest and tell you that even though Dr. Chung has cut me off from more IVF, and I'm at peace as an adoptive mom, I still think about going back into treatment. I am not sure I can accept the fact that I can never carry a pregnancy to term.

I know way too much about infertility, its causes and treatments. I have more things wrong with me than most people do, and I have gone through more tests and treatments than most people. There is nothing in this book that I don't know about firsthand. From tests to surgeries, to treatment, to pregnancy, to miscarriage, to pursuing adoption, child-free living, or using a surrogate, I have been there and done that. I hope what I've learned along the way can help you.

# 2

# Surviving the Infertility Roller Coaster

## THIS DEFINITELY AIN'T A VACATION AT DISNEY WORLD

There are three basic things that you need to know about surviving the infertility roller coaster. I discovered this the hard way. Follow these three basic rules, and your experience with assisted reproductive technologies (ART) may be a little easier. These rules work. Modify them if you want to make them work better for you as an individual, but seriously, *use them.*

## Rule #1
## Remember: Start with a Clean Slate Whenever Possible

The first thing that I had to accept about infertility treatment is that it's a process, and it can be a very *long* process at that. There are, however, ways to speed it up, and I've learned that a lot of it has to do with making smart choices at the outset. (We'll talk about smart choices in chapter 7.) But even when I made choices that moved me closer to my goal— becoming pregnant—I still had to deal with this head trip I was on. I needed to be pregnant *now!*

As far as I was concerned, by the time I met Dr. Motormouth (not to mention Dr. Chung), I'd been trying to conceive for three years, and I had to get pregnant *that instant*. Once you start treatment, however, you need to forget everything you've done to have a baby before you walk through your RE's door for tests and treatment or your adoption agency's doors. You need a clean slate.

Trust me on this. Forget that you've been trying for two months, twelve years, or however long you've been at it. I know this sounds impossible. All that matters in your life is getting pregnant *now*, and you have no patience left. None, zip, zero. You want to be pregnant yesterday!

It's not going to happen. There are tests and more tests, not to mention phone calls and office visits with the doctor, before your first cycle using ART even begins. High-tech infertility treatments like in vitro fertilization (IVF) can increase your odds of conceiving per cycle to those of the most fertile twenty-year-old or (at some clinics and with some technologies) to those of the three most fertile twenty-year-olds. But it's going to take some time—and a lot of emotional energy—before you've got those odds. If you're adopting, you've got applications, home-study visits, INS forms, and/or adoptive parent profiles to complete before your international referral comes or a birth family selects you. Wipe your memory slate clean and pretend you just started trying to have a baby. I know this isn't easy to do.

In fact, each time you get more information about what is causing your infertility or you try something new and different, wipe the slate clean and pretend you're starting from scratch. I have done this several times, and it really helps. The last time I did this was after my second IVF cycle (which, if you recall, followed four IUIs, three major surgeries, and more than four years of trying to conceive) when I was diagnosed with that blood-clotting disorder. Once we had this diagnosis, Dr. Chung felt that I might never before have had a real chance of getting pregnant. I was thrilled to have an answer for why I wasn't getting pregnant. My other cycles hadn't had a chance. Suddenly, it was like we were starting over.

When we were starting that third IVF cycle, Charlie reminded me of the Clean Slate Rule. I thought he was insane. How could I forget about all that we'd been through? But I did manage to wipe the slate clean. Each day of that IVF cycle I reminded myself that this was my first real chance to conceive. Whenever I got scared or nervous, I reminded myself this was a whole new ball game, a new chance, a first chance. Wiping the slate clean really does work. I got through my third IVF cycle, and I got pregnant!

## Rule #2
## Remember: The Infertility Roller Coaster Is Horrible for Everyone

The second thing I had to accept about dealing with infertility and using ART is that this roller coaster is as frightening and exhilarating as anything at a Six Flags amusement park. Whether you're going for initial screening tests, waiting to get on the wait list at a famous clinic, taking fertility drugs, or enduring the two-week wait to find out if you're pregnant, the highs and lows are going to hit you hard. This is normal. Tell your husband to be prepared for crying jags that seem to come out of nowhere and last for days, and warn him that you may turn into what Charlie fondly calls an RLB (raving lunatic bitch) at the drop of a fork.

At the beginning of my experience with ART, I went shopping at the local Big K. I was tired and depressed, and I was completely unprepared for what happened when I got to the store. Something about the size—this Big K is *big*—was completely overwhelming, and I started to

Ladies and gentlemen, welcome to the Infertility Roller Coaster. Please make sure your safety restraint is securely locked, and keep your arms and hands inside the vehicle at all times. Do not attempt to disembark the roller coaster until it has come to a complete stop.

panic. I started sobbing hysterically. Soon I was completely paralyzed by grief and depression. I was standing in the Martha Stewart linens section losing my mind—not to mention rapidly dehydrating—and I had no idea why. No one had told me that the side effects of Clomid, which was being used during one of my ART cycles, include mood swings and depression. I was paralyzed for days. I did manage to get out of the store and into my car. God only knows what all those Kmart shoppers thought of me! Charlie swore we were stopping all ART, I freaked out at the thought of not continuing treatment, and then boom, it went away. That was my introduction to the roller coaster. (By the way, I've had friends who experienced absolutely no side effects from Clomid. *Go figure!*)

Soon after I recovered from the Big K incident, I found out—during an ultrasound—that Dr. Motormouth was leaving my clinic. I could continue treatment at her new office three hours from my house, or she could refer me to another doctor in the clinic (who might or might not be on my insurance plan). I was stunned. Things only got worse. The ultrasound she was performing as she was telling me about her wonderful new job revealed a cyst on one of my ovaries. In between breaths about the new job, she told me the cyst might mean that she would have to cancel my cycle, and oh yeah, there was also a polyp in my uterine cavity that was growing rather rapidly and might need to be surgically removed. My head was spinning. I had gone to the clinic for routine blood work and an ultrasound and found that I had no doctor, I had a cyst and possibly wouldn't be able to cycle that month, and I might need surgery. Dr. Motormouth sped out of the ultrasound room after reminding me that I would get my usual afternoon phone call letting me know whether I could start the cycle (it would depend on my estradiol, also known as my estrogen or E2 level, discussed in chapter 11).

I went home, cried, waited for my phone call, and cried some more. Wait to do another cycle? *Wait?* I couldn't wait five seconds let alone another month! *More* surgery? I couldn't face more surgery! I had no doctor! How would I survive this? All I wanted was my chance at conception for the month. The hours ticked by as I waited for my phone call.

Finally, at six o'clock that night, the nurse called and told me I could

**A word to the wise:** | Time goes really slowly when you're in infertility treatment. Start thinking about your life in components of hours rather than days. Mastering the art of surviving hour to hour will serve you well in the long run. You can start by making a list of things you can do to distract and soothe yourself while you wait. Try a cup of tea, a walk to Starbucks for a decaf mocha (with your cell phone of course, in case your RE's office calls), knitting or needlepoint, renting movies, reading, yoga or meditation, or anything else that will help you pass the time and stay sane.

start my injections and my cycle that night. *Woohoo!* My E2 level was normal, so the cyst wasn't something to worry about. As for the polyp, my new doctor would make the decision about any surgery. The nurse suggested I make an appointment with my new RE as soon as possible, because he had a waiting list.

"Excuse me, did you say 'waiting list'? I have to *wait* to see him?" I practically screamed at the nurse. "I am already a patient of the clinic, I am already receiving treatment, it's not my fault my doctor is leaving the clinic, I've been trying to conceive for three years, I am *not capable of waiting!*"

And so went one day in my life as an infertility patient. Unanticipated rapid descents, sharp turns, frighteningly fast escalating climbs, and nauseating swoops. Now, just so I don't completely scare you, please know that I also have had IUI and IVF cycles in which everything went beautifully, and I never lost it. My advice, however: expect the roller coaster to be brutal; it is brutal for everyone at one time or another (the woman who says it's not hard is lying). At the very least you will be prepared (I wasn't), and once in a while you might even be pleasantly surprised. The roller coaster is a little less frightening if you know that: (1) everyone has bad days; (2) this stuff is really hard for everyone to deal with; and, (3) for every bad day, there is a day that will be better.

**A word to the wise:** | As difficult as it may be for you to believe, your RE/clinic has a patient who has been trying to conceive longer than you have. Pointing out to your nurse/doctor how long you have been trying to conceive and how little patience you have does *not* work. In the world of infertility—and elsewhere—the reasonable person is far more likeable than the hysterical, impatient, and demanding one. You probably won't get better medical care just by being easy to deal with, but having a good relationship with your doctor and nurse can ease a lot of tense moments. You want your nurse and doctor to like working with you. Do not vent in their direction unless absolutely necessary!

## Rule #3
## Remember: Treating Infertility Is Like Peeling an Onion

The third thing I discovered during my fertility treatment is that dealing with infertility is a lot like peeling an onion: There are a lot of layers. Nothing ever seems to be straightforward. You fix one problem, you discover another; you do two IVF cycles, then have to have more surgery; you get pregnant, then you miscarry. It always seems like you are taking two steps forward and then three steps back. Diagnosing and treating infertility is an incredibly frustrating experience. And it makes you cry. You just have to keep peeling the layers away, even though you're crying so hard you can't see how many more layers there are to peel and how much smaller the onion is getting.

With an onion, you know that in the end you will have peeled all of it and there will be nothing left; mission accomplished! With infertility, however, you don't know the outcome, or think you don't know the outcome. You actually have the power to determine the outcome (something we will discuss later in this book). You are *not* a passive passenger on this roller coaster. It is your body and your life. You can decide when and if you think you need a different doctor, when and if you need to take a break, when and if you've had enough. If it's a baby you want, it's a baby you ultimately will get. It's always your choice. But often this gets forgotten when you hit a particularly frustrating time during your treatment, and all you can do is cry.

For those days when you have the greatest sense of despair, try to look at your infertility treatment as a process similar to peeling an onion. As the tears fall, remember the layers are falling away, and you will, eventually, reach your goal.

And when you're crying so hard you can't see that the onion is getting smaller and you're indeed making progress, it's not a bad idea to let someone else into the kitchen to take over the peeling. It is your body, but you cannot solve your infertility problems by yourself. You need your RE to design the treatment protocol that's right for you, your partner's love and support (not to mention, probably, his sperm), and the help of technicians and nurses. Each one of these people will take a turn peeling so that you may achieve your goal. When the going gets tough—really, really tough—remember that there are other people there to help you.

So, when you have just come off a particularly bumpy section of your ride on the infertility roller coaster, remember my three basic rules for survival.

- Remember to start with a clean slate whenever possible.

- Remember that the infertility roller coaster is brutal, and everyone has a hard time surviving the ride.

- Remember that treating infertility is a lot like peeling an onion; there is an end, even if you can't see it through the tears.

These rules help me see my infertility with a new perspective and give me a little more hope.

# 3

# Finding a Good Reproductive Endocrinologist or Fertility Clinic

YOU BETTER LIKE YOUR DOCTOR, BECAUSE YOU'RE
ABOUT TO BUY HER A NEW BMW

There are a couple of different types of doctors who treat infertility. Since most women hate going to the doctor (especially if it involves stirrups and a speculum), you're going to want to find the right doctor as quickly as possible and save yourself unnecessary exams. Initially, most women seek treatment from their gynecologist. However, it's probably a better idea to see a reproductive endocrinologist, or RE. REs are gynecologists who have received highly specialized training in infertility and the female endocrine (hormone) system as it pertains to reproduction. Reproductive endocrinologists are usually board certified—meaning they've taken a very difficult, specialized exam—in treating reproductive disorders that can cause infertility. Gynecologists (GYNs)—board certified or not—who specialize in infertility don't have this training. Even the best GYN cannot treat you as effectively and quickly as an RE can. Don't waste precious time; go see an RE.

You cannot just assume your infertility lies with your reproductive system. You need to get your husband or partner checked out by a urologist. Urologists specialize in dealing with the urinary tract system and male physiology. Some urologists receive specialized training in infertility and deal exclusively with male-factor infertility. There are treatments for certain kinds of male-factor infertility (see chapter 6 for more information on male-factor infertility) that may enable you to get pregnant without the use of assisted reproductive technologies like IVF (in vitro fertilization). If you're having trouble finding a urologist, ask your GYN or RE for a referral. Okay, enough of a detour into men's stuff. Let's talk about finding *you* the right doctor.

I recommend putting together a list of physicians who you might want to see and then interviewing all of them. This takes time and money—two things that are probably in short supply right now. But finding the right doctor is extremely important, and the only way to do this is to meet the candidates, talk to them, and judge their capabilities and bedside manner.

Fertility treatment is a multibillion-dollar industry. Making matters worse, most infertility treatments are paid for in cash, up front. As a result, there are a lot of bad doctors—*quacks*—out there trying to make a quick buck. And even among good, reputable practices, fertility specialists are not created equal. The world of infertility treatment involves cutting-edge technologies and constantly advancing medical frontiers. It is imperative that you find a doctor who is on top of all the developments in her field. Would you go to an oncologist (cancer doctor) or a neurologist (brain doctor) who was using therapies and treatments that were state-of-the-art two or three years ago but have been replaced by new, better, more effective treatments? Of course not! So why do it now? You're spending huge amounts of time and money, investing a ton of emotional and physical energy, and trying to create a new life, your *child*. You won't know if the RE you want to go to is at the top of her game unless you speak to a couple of doctors and compare their levels of expertise.

Having a doctor that meets your needs also is extremely important when you're dealing with an area of your life that is so emotionally charged. This experience has been hard enough for you so far and, quite honestly, it's only going to get more demanding (that's really an understatement). You need a doctor who you trust, respect, and like.

Trust me, you're going to think about your RE constantly and share some very emotional times with her. This doctor will have the power to shatter your emotional well-being in one sentence ("I'm sorry but . . ."), and lift you to the heavens in two words ("You're pregnant!"). This doctor will see more of your vagina than your significant other will be seeing (trust me on this) and is going to play a bigger role in your life than any other doctor, except (hopefully) your obstetrician. And let's not forget the other not-so-little part of this equation: you're about to spend tens of thousands of your (or your insurance company's) money with this doctor. You don't want to feel that you just bought the world's biggest jerk (or biggest quack) a new BMW. Make sure you like her and that she has the right kind of practice style—bedside manner—for your personality.

It was only through comparisons between doctors that I was able to learn what was important to me and what I was going to need from my RE both personally and professionally. After being horrified by dirty exam room floors, outdated ultrasound equipment, doctors who'd never heard of my blood-clotting disorder or the treatment for it, and who kept me waiting for over an hour and then were dismissive and arrogant or downright rude, I realized I needed a state-of-the-art practice and a really compassionate doctor who was up on the latest research, treatments, and techniques: the three S's, (1) state-of-the-art, (2) sympathetic, and (3) smart.

To do this, you've gotta interview doctors. There just is no other way. Whether you're new to treatment and just getting started finding a doctor, or you've been through some treatment and aren't grooving on your doctor, or you aren't getting good results from your treatment and want to see if you've got more options, make a list of potential candidates for your business. Your list is going to be very important, so draw it up carefully.

Start by contacting RESOLVE, the American Infertility Association (AIA), or the American Society for Reproductive Medicine (ASRM)—all these organizations are listed in the Resources section at the back of the book—for a referral to an RE or a good fertility clinic (and don't forget about getting your husband in to see a urologist). These organizations have prescreened lists of physicians who specialize in treating infertility in your area of the country. These lists can save you time. You know these doctors are likely to be good if a big organization like RESOLVE or ASRM has put them on their "approved" list. If you have any friends that had trouble getting pregnant, ask them where they went for treatment (they might even turn out to be a great source of support for you). If you've already been receiving treatment and know what's wrong with you, these organizations can help you compile a list of REs or urologists who specialize in treating your specific type of infertility.

The Web is another great place to go to get information, but you need to be very choosy about the sites you visit and the sources of the information on which you rely. Patients you meet on-line can give you great feedback about a particular doctor or clinic. Relying on their information about your medical condition can be far more dangerous. You have no way of knowing the level of intelligence of the person you are communicating with, or her degree of understanding of her condition and how she's being treated. Unless you know the woman you're talking to on the Web, take the medical information she gives you with a *big* grain of salt.

You need to be similarly wary with respect to Web sites. Some offer articles written by doctors, bulletin boards on which doctors answer patients' questions, and bulletin boards on which you can chat with other patients. These can be great resources for you. Beware, however; many of the bulletin boards monitored by doctors are marketing tools for the physician who answers questions on that board. Some of these physicians use experimental therapies that may serve no benefit to you (or anyone else for that matter).

This is not necessarily the time to become a human guinea pig (I've been there and done that, and trust me, avoid it if you can!) nor is it the time to go off the deep end into uber-alternative treatment. I heard of one woman who decided to try some new therapy based on lunar cycles (you know, the transits of the moon!) that she heard about on a Web bulletin board. I'm all for alternative medicine, but there's a not-too-fine line between something like acupuncture and medical treatment based on houses of the moon (Nancy Reagan may disagree, but she wasn't trying to have a baby). Talk to your doctor before you take advice you receive from someone on the Internet. She's intimately familiar with your medical history and condition (we hope) and can help make sure that the experimental therapy doesn't jeopardize your health or the success of the rest of your infertility treatment.

You also need to be very wary of a doctor that never sees you but merely reviews your medical history based solely on what you tell him in an E-mail and prescribes a treatment. That is unprofessional, dangerous, and (in my legal opinion), borders on malpractice (old habits die hard; I guess I'm a lawyer to the core). Many of the more reputable doctors who post on Web sites require that you submit a *written medical history* from your doctor and obtain—at the very least—a phone consultation. Sometimes they even want to talk to your RE; this is a *good* sign that you're not dealing with a quack! In some states it is illegal to give medical advice via E-mail or over the Internet. Make sure to do your homework about the doctor and the therapy before you spend money and invest emotional energy in something that may not work. Do you really want to buy this quack a BMW?

Remember, reproductive medicine is a *consumer business*. You are the consumer. And the old consumer adage, "Buyer beware" applies just as much to reproductive medicine as it does to any other consumer industry. This is another reason you'll want to be very careful compiling your list of doctors and why you want to interview them and compare their bedside manner and competence.

Before you start interviewing and picking doctors, however, there are two basic things you need to know: (1) what you need and want in a doctor and (2) how successful the doctor or clinic is at treating couples, especially those with your medical issues (if you know ahead of time what they are). If you're needy (and by the way, that's okay to admit), you need a doctor who's okay with patients who require a lot of her time. If you want quick and businesslike, you shouldn't have a doctor who's always trying to hold your hand. If you have a busy job, you can't be spending two hours waiting to see her.

Start thinking about all the doctors you've seen in your life and make a list of those who you liked and disliked and why. Make a list of your priorities before you start calling doctors up and interviewing them. Here are some things to think about as you create your list.

*Do the doctors you like tend to be very businesslike and no-nonsense, or are they very compassionate and take the time to listen to you complain about work?*

Think about getting bad news from your RE. Do you want the doctor to break the news gently and be sympathetic and listen while you cry, or do you want someone who's going to tell you in a no-nonsense manner that your treatment isn't working (or whatever horrible thing you never want to imagine hearing)? I've had both kinds of REs. Dr. Motormouth was no-nonsense (to the point of being rude) and Dr. Chung is about as compassionate as they get. Let me tell you, I'd rather hear bad news from a compassionate doctor than one who makes you feel like she just wants to get rid of you because you're ruining her success rates.

*Do you like to know what's going on from a medical standpoint and have someone speak to you as if you have an advanced degree? Or do you want someone who can explain things to you in a more simplistic manner?*

I need someone who can do both. I've got a pretty good head for understanding medical stuff (if you haven't figured that out yet, you will later in the book), but there've been times after a miscarriage when I was so distraught that I needed someone to explain to me what was going on and what was about to happen as if I were in kindergarten.

*Do you hate long waits in a waiting room?*

Tell me about it! Sometimes this is unavoidable, but you can look for responsive nurses' stations or receptionists who will move you ahead of other people on the day you-absolutely-have-to-get-out-of-there-and-can't-wait-another-minute-or-you'll-lose-your-job. Current magazines or newspapers in the waiting room are helpful (there's nothing worse than a waiting room with last year's *National Geographic*), or a quiet waiting room so you can do work or read. A courtesy phone is good, so you can call whomever you were supposed to meet half an hour ago without incurring a charge on your cell phone. Sometimes waiting in a doctor's office can be okay; there are times I enjoy being left alone to page through *Cosmo*, but none of us want to do it every day.

### *Do you need to have a doctor return your calls, or is it okay if a nurse calls you back to answer your question?*

Believe it or not, this can be a big deal. You may think it's okay to speak to a nurse, but then one day you have a question only the doctor can answer. You wait hours and sometimes even days to get an answer or instructions. Some doctors return phone calls themselves (albeit at *weird* hours of the day) and it might be more important to you to speak to her instead of the nurse. Personally, I would rather get the results faster from a nurse and then wait (not so patiently) for the doctor to get back to me with more detailed information. But I know some women who absolutely insist on speaking with their RE and *only* their RE.

### *Do you prefer male physicians to female physicians?*

This is a no-brainer for most of us. Unfortunately, however, most REs are men. If you don't mind men doctors checking you out down there, then it won't be a problem for you. If it is, you may have to look a little harder to find a good female RE in your area.

Same thing goes with age. If you have a preference for a younger RE, this shouldn't be an issue for you; most REs are under forty-five (it is, after all, a fairly new area of medical science). Some are older and more established in their practices. However, given their "advanced age" (I just had to find a way to get back at these ageist REs!) they may not see many patients (they tend to be the pioneers in the field) and may have long waiting lists. Speaking of waiting lists, the really young REs are generally just starting out in practice and may not have a long wait list. If you can find one who trained at a great clinic, she may be better trained and up on the latest treatments and theories than some of the older guys and be able to see you sooner.

*Do you like to have a doctor with an office close to your home or your office?*

I can't answer this question for you, as I live in a major metropolitan area and had several preeminent fertility centers to choose from. That said, however, there are some less well-known clinics in my region that have far lower success rates, and I was constantly surprised at the number of women who chose to get treated at the local clinic that was fifteen minutes from their home, when for another thirty minutes (total commute forty-five minutes, with traffic) they could see the best of the best. But I'll talk more about distinguishing between the good and the bad in fertility clinics in a minute. I'll chalk this one up to convenience; and sometimes having something be conveniently located cannot be overlooked.

*Do you care whether your doctor is in network with your insurance plan, or will you go to a doctor that is highly recommended to you but does not accept insurance or is not on your insurance plan?*

This can be very important later on when you're dealing with finances, but initially it's worth assessing your need to go to the best possible doctor regardless of insurance. This might be the time to indulge your preference for the best medical care. I grew up in a place with some of the best medical care available on earth and the old-fashioned indemnity insurance plans (no co-pays, no networks), so when someone got sick, we got recommendations from other doctors and went to the best doctor around. I don't believe in messing around with medical care, and until all this started—and infertility treatments started draining my bank account with alarming speed—I didn't care whether I was getting 80 percent reimbursed at the usual and customary rate (see chapter 9) or 100 percent

**A word to the wise:** | Make sure to send *all of your medical records* well in advance of the appointment to interview a doctor. There's nothing worse than sitting there wasting the limited amount of time you've got to talk to this doctor while she's reading up on your medical history, or feeling angry and frustrated that she can't answer your questions because you've forgotten to send the one record that is most important for her analysis of your condition and prognosis. While some doctors may wait to read your medical records even if you've sent them weeks in advance—this might be a tip-off that this doctor isn't thorough enough for your taste—at least you know you've tried. And if it does happen and it pisses you off, confront the doctor about it. If they have the medical records, most physicians do take the time to read up on potential new patients before they walk through the consultation doors.

with the $5 co-pay. Charlie grew up with the nasty ol' HMO and really balked at the idea of going to anyone who was out of network. Trying to pick a doctor with these two different paradigms was a battle in and of itself.

And finally (although this list is by no means all-inclusive):

*What qualities in a doctor make you trust her and have confidence in her?*

I'd go with your gut instinct on this. Sometimes you just *know* when someone is right for you. But if you have seen doctors that you loved and seen some you hated, try to figure out what it was about the bad ones that made them *bad*.

Once you have determined what your needs are, you're going to have to meet the doctor to determine whether you've got a good match.

Here are some sample questions you might want to ask the doctor to help you figure out if she will meet your needs. For your convenience, I've reprinted this list in the Appendix without the discussion that follows here. Feel free to photocopy the list and take it with you when you're interviewing REs).

*How much time on average do you allocate to your appointments with patients? How strictly do you follow this schedule?*

Most doctors, especially those with busy practices or those restricted by managed care, can only give you fifteen minutes, and that has to include an exam. Ain't much time to ask questions and get thorough answers, is it? Reproductive practices, while not usually subject to the hassles of HMOs (if you find a reproductive group in your HMO, please let me know!) tend to have hefty patient loads. This either means you never get a good conversation with your doctor or she's perpetually backed up. I have seen doctors who tried to deal with this by allocating twenty minutes to each patient for regular visits, and longer for patients experiencing complications like a miscarriage. Scheduling must be a nightmare for these doctors, but it works well for patients.

If your problem is that you've got a busy schedule (who doesn't?), find out if the practice has early or late hours to accommodate you. Find out whether you can expect to see your RE every visit during a treatment cycle or whether you will see a nurse, technician, or other doctor (physician's assistant, medical resident, or fellow). Many times your RE will handle specific appointments, but during a cycle someone else will handle the daily monitoring.

*Do you prefer patients who ask detailed questions about treatment, diagnosis, or symptoms?*

Doctors are surprisingly honest about this, and many of them prefer patients who understand their medical condition and the treatment for it. Many women never ask questions (something I don't advocate in this book). If you're going to want to be on autopilot with your RE, make sure she isn't going to offer complicated explanations when you don't want her to.

*Are you available by phone, fax, or E-mail?*

Sometimes a doctor prefers to receive or respond to nonemergency questions by E-mail or fax rather than the phone. This enables your RE to assess the question and think about it before responding to your query. It's also a great way to deal with the follow-up question you forgot to ask when you had your RE on the phone.

*What time of day do you usually return phone calls?*

Find out when this is. If you're not available during her phone hour, you need to have an alternate system in place for communicating with her.

The next and final thing to consider when choosing an RE is to evaluate the level of technical competence of the physicians or facilities you're looking at. You want to know whether you're going to have a good chance at getting pregnant with this RE, regardless of her bedside manner.

I've interviewed at different-sized clinics and have spoken with my friends who have cycled at a variety of places. From everything I can tell—although there are notable exceptions—you have far better odds of conceiving a baby and carrying to term if you cycle at one of the big, really outstanding fertility centers. Maybe I'm just biased to name brands or something (I'm sure Charlie will agree with me here), but sometimes bigger and better-known really is better! We're not buying a pair of jeans where any Gap will do; we're making a baby and contemplating spending tens of thousands of dollars! Remember the old adage: you get what you pay for!

There are some outstanding small clinics in the United States and elsewhere around the world where you have great chances of getting pregnant. Choosing a smaller, less well-known center doesn't mean you won't get pregnant right away, and it might be a more pleasant experience for you to cycle in a more intimate environment (big clinics can make you feel like you're a number, not a person). But keep in mind that, for the most part, bigger research-oriented clinics have better laboratory facilities (they have more money to buy the latest state-of-the-art equipment), better physicians and staff (it's competitive to work in these clinics; you're getting the best of the best), and better success (because they try new and different things and are constantly evaluating the state of medical knowledge and technology). You need to consider the competence of the lab your RE relies on just as much as you want to find the right RE.

You want the best embryologist (the person who takes care of your embryos) and andrologist (the person who takes care of your husband's sperm) money can buy. I can't tell you the number of women I've spoken to who cycled repeatedly with a less than state-of-the-art team of lab technicians and equipment and were told that they didn't get pregnant because their eggs or sperm (or both) weren't up to par. When they switched to clinics with better labs, they had absolutely no problem achieving pregnancy and were told—point-blank—that their prior problems had been due to poor handling or management of their eggs and/or sperm by the lab at their old clinic.

A good embryologist and andrologist can help save a cycle that may be compromised by a poor stimulation protocol. Mediocre eggs and poor sperm can still achieve a pregnancy if the embryologist and/or andrologist are sufficiently proficient at recognizing instances where ICSI (where the sperm is injected into the egg to assist fertilization), rescue ICSI (same procedure done after standard fertilization techniques have failed), or assisted hatching (where a hole is drilled into the shell of the fertilized egg to help it hatch out of its shell and implant in the uterine wall) are warranted and are successful at performing these procedures (see chapters 6 and 12 for more on these techniques). It's terribly frustrating to waste time and money at a clinic that has a lab that actually impedes your chances of conceiving.

Here are some sample questions to help you find out about the lab (once again, I've listed these questions in the Appendix in case you want to take them with you to your RE's office).

*Is the clinic affiliated with or part of a research- or academic-based medical center like a hospital?*

Research- or academic-based facilities often have more money to use to purchase equipment and hire staff. Their interest lies not only in getting you pregnant but in developing new techniques to help couples achieve pregnancy, and in order to do this, they need state-of-the-art facilities.

*Is the embryology lab located at the hospital?*

Generally, labs in hospitals are more sophisticated than those located in a doctor's private office or stand-alone facility (although there are notable exceptions). If you're interested, some clinics will give you a tour of the lab.

*Is the embryologist an M.D. or a board-certified Ph.D., known in the industry as a high-complexity clinical laboratory director?*

The latter qualification is the bare minimum you want in an embryologist. Ask the RE you're interviewing this question, although you also can ask to meet with the embryologist as well.

*Has the embryologist or andrologist been responsible for discovering or improving any techniques or technologies?*

*Does s/he publish articles on the clinic's research?*

There are a couple of centers on the East Coast of the United States that have world-famous embryologists and andrologists. They publish textbooks, write articles, and design new techniques to assist fertilization. You don't necessarily need to go to a fertility clinic with this level of expertise, but if there are good people in your area, you owe it to yourself to find out about them.

*How often is the embryology lab cleaned?*

About every three to four months should be sufficient.

*Who is the andrologist?*

Again, examine credentials and find out how long the andrologist has been practicing, where he was trained, whether he has published articles or developed any new techniques.

When assessing the expertise of the clinic, you might want to ask the following questions:

*How many IVF egg retrievals and embryo transfers does the clinic perform per week?*

At the bigger centers the answer to this question may be thirty or more retrievals per week for an individual doctor where the clinic overall performs around one hundred per week; smaller centers may be in the single digits per week for the doctor *and* the clinic. One woman I know interviewed with a doctor who was proud of the fact that he did eighty retrievals and transfers a year. This is great for him, but some of the bigger centers have doctors who do that many in two weeks. What does this tell you about their relative experience performing these procedures?

*How many embryos does the clinic transfer to a patient in your age group and/or with your medical condition?*

Most clinics and REs have guidelines for embryo transfer with IVF (for example, three to four eggs for women aged thirty-four and under) but are willing to work with you if you aren't comfortable with their policies.

*What types of procedures are available to your patients?*

Get a detailed list from your RE or clinic. A lab that doesn't offer and regularly perform ICSI, assisted hatching, frozen embryo transfers, and blastocyst transfers *isn't worth your time*. You also want a clinic that has a good coculture program. Standard culture programs may not be as helpful to you if you have egg and embryo quality issues as a clinic offering an advanced coculture program. Because these techniques can make the difference between an unsuccessful cycle and a successful one; *you must have these as options in your treatment plan* (see chapters 7 and 12 for more information).

*How many frozen embryo transfers do they perform per year?*

The more the better! Although this is not necessarily a goal of IVF cycles, it's good to know that you have the option of using frozen embryos if you wind up with too many to use for your fresh cycle (lucky you!).

*What are the criteria for freezing eggs?*

Clinics that are very fussy about freezing eggs may not be right for you; clinics that aren't fussy about what they freeze may not be right for you.

*What is the protocol for frozen embryo transfers (FETs)?*

Does the clinic only do natural cycle FETs, or do they prefer to control you with medication? Program—or medically controlled—FETs tend to be more successful but also not as relaxed as natural cycle FETs.

*Does the clinic do blastocyst transfers?*

I talk about what this is in detail in chapter 12, but for right now all you need to know is that it is a relatively new IVF technique of transferring more-developed embryos that are stronger, healthier, and more likely to result in a pregnancy. Only the more sophisticated labs are able to provide this service to you. Because this is one of those techniques that should be an option for you, a lab/clinic that doesn't offer blastocyst transfer is not ideal.

### What are the clinic's criteria for performing blastocyst transfers?

Some clinics only perform blastocyst transfers on very young patients, while others prefer to make it their goal for all patients. If you're at a clinic that makes blastocyst transfer their goal for all patients, you might be disappointed (and feel like a failure) if your embryos don't qualify for this kind of transfer (see chapter 12).

### How many blastocyst transfers do they perform per year?

The more the better, if you ask me.

Find out everything you can about the lab, and go with the best lab you can find. It's worth it in the long run.

Some questions to ask the RE you're interviewing to help assess her competence and approach to treating you (and compare it to what other REs may tell you) are:

*Where did you go to medical school?*

*Where did you do your residency; where did you train?*

*Are you board certified?*

*How long have you been practicing reproductive medicine?*

*Have you published any articles?*

*Do you give lectures? Do you travel frequently to give lectures?*

*Do you have any specific expertise, for example treating endometriosis or polycystic ovarian syndrome?*

Watch out for doctors who are really aggressive. Aggressive REs take risks with patient care in an effort to improve their success rates. This puts you at risk for having a high-order multiple pregnancy (see chapter 12) or developing complications like OHSS (page 146). Here are some questions that can help you assess her aggressiveness.

### How many eggs do you seek to recruit for IVF patients?

Most conservative (read safe) clinics shoot for ten to twelve as the ideal number of eggs to recruit. The ultimate result (how many eggs are produced during an IVF cycle) is dependent on the individual patient, but a question like this can help you determine how aggressive your RE is.

### What percentage of your patients experience OHSS (ovarian hyperstimulation syndrome, discussed in greater detail in chapter 7)?

Most conservative clinics do not want to risk having patients develop OHSS. A good conservative rate is 10 to 15 percent. Anything more than that, and the clinic you're considering may be dangerously aggressive.

### What are your criteria for canceling a patient's cycle?

You want to know ahead of time if your RE or fertility clinic cancels roughly half of all IVF cycles due to complications. This may be due to their conservatism and may be a good thing in the long run (better safe than sorry), but you want to know ahead of time what your odds are for getting to retrieval and transfer.

### How would you recommend I start treatment?

Find out if the RE thinks you should start with IUIs or move straight to IVF, and find out why. (I'll talk about the merits of starting with one or the other treatment in chapter 7.)

*What types of protocols do you use?*

You want the answer here to be that it depends on the individual woman and her condition.

*What type of protocol would you recommend for me?*

*What do you think my prognosis is?*

This is perhaps the toughest question to ask, because you're afraid of the answer. But you *must* ask it of each physician you interview. If there's consensus among the doctors that you have an excellent prognosis, that's wonderful and you should be excited. It's tougher when each doctor tells you something different or has a different assessment of how you should approach treatment and why. If you're choosing between two REs who have differing opinions of how you should get started (one says IUI while the other suggests IVF, or one proposes surgery before treatment and one says you should get started right away), call and ask follow-up questions. Ask them to assess the other approach to treatment and tell you why they recommend something different.

Getting answers to these questions ensures that you are an educated consumer and can make the best decision possible when picking an RE or clinic. The competition for your business is out of control, and doctors promise things they cannot deliver in order to get your business. In an article in the *New York Times* ("Fertility Inc.: Clinics Race to Lure Clients," the *New York Times*, January 1, 2002, F1) writer Gina Kolata exposed a very dirty little secret. Many REs send local OB-GYNs and other medical professionals on vacations, out for fancy dinners, or give them other valuable gifts in exchange for referring business. Yep, your trusted OB-GYN may have referred you to a particular RE because he really enjoyed his gift trip to the Caribbean, not because of that RE's expertise. It's one thing to offer special financing arrangements to patients like shared-risk and money-back programs to help get your business (chapter 9); it's another to pay or bribe someone to refer business.

Other marketing tactics to watch out for include inflating success rates or success rates presented in misleading ways. In fact, one of the first things you need to know when you're evaluating a particular clinic is its success rates. And you'll need to understand how in vitro programs characterize their success in order to get a realistic idea of how likely you are to get pregnant.

## Making Sense of Success Rates

Understanding success rates is really hard; don't feel frustrated if you feel you need a Ph.D. in statistical mathematics to understand this stuff.

First, find out whether your doctor or clinic officially reports statistics either to the Centers for Disease Control (CDC) or the Society for Assisted Reproductive Technologies (SART), a special division of the American Society for Reproductive Medicine. You also want to know whether those statistics are independently audited by a certified public accountant. Many centers publish audited statistics; these are more reliable than statistics that have not been reviewed for accuracy. Both CDC and SART publish annual reports of various clinics' success rates, and you can consider these reports and their statistics accurate and reliable. In the Resources section, I've given you a link to the CDC's Web site of annual ART statistics.

These reports are broken down into age-based categories, so you can determine your likely success rate based on your age. Sometimes you can even find reports broken down by condition or diagnosis, although these tend not to be published. If you are curious, ask your doctor or clinic if they have statistics for women with your condition (endometriosis, premature ovarian failure, PCOS, etc.). The pregnancy rate is the success rate. Makes sense, right? This is what you want to look at.

Make sure you know how your clinic defines its success/pregnancy rates. It might be based on the total number of transfers performed, per embryo transferred (the number of embryos actually transferred will be higher than the number of transfers performed; most clinics transfer about three embryos in each transfer procedure performed), the number of egg retrievals performed (which will be higher than the number of transfers, as not all women who undergo retrievals will have embryos to transfer), or per the number of women in the program (even higher than both the other numbers, because not all women in the program will make it to retrieval, let alone transfer).

Statistics based on a per-transfer calculation refer to an average success rate based on each embryo transfer procedure performed. This method of calculating success slightly inflates a clinic's success rates because it doesn't include those cycles where a woman fails to get to embryo transfer. Because her cycle was canceled before retrieval (because she failed to produce eggs or her eggs failed to fertilize after retrieval), she never made it to embryo transfer and thus her cycle failure is not reflected in the clinic's overall success rate. Had her cycle (and its lack of a resulting pregnancy) been included in the statistics, the success rate would have been lower.

If the statistic is based on the total number of women cycling in the program, the clinic's success rates will be further inflated because this method doesn't tell you how many cycles it took those women to get pregnant. This doesn't tell you anything about the likelihood that you'll get pregnant in any one cycle.

Perhaps the fairest way to calculate success rates—and the best way for you to figure out how likely you are to get pregnant during an IVF cycle—is to measure success based on the number of egg retrievals performed. Once a woman gets to retrieval, she is officially a candidate for IVF, whether or not her eggs actually fertilize or grow sufficiently to be transferred back to her uterus. If her eggs fail to fertilize or her embryos arrest (die) before transfer, her failed cycle is still reflected in the clinic's statistics and gives you a more realistic sense of how many women (what percentage of patients undergoing the procedure) really get pregnant.

You also need to consider whether a given success rate reflects chemical or clinical pregnancy rates or live-birth rates. Each of these pregnancy rates measures the pregnancy from a different point in time, and with a different statistical chance of the pregnancy carrying to term.

A chemical pregnancy is one that is detected by blood tests. It is the earliest stages of a pregnancy, so it still has a significant chance of resulting in miscarriage. A clinical pregnancy, which is confirmed by the presence of a heartbeat on ultrasound, has progressed a little further. Once a heartbeat is detected, the chances of the pregnancy miscarrying drop significantly. Because the incidence of early miscarriage is so high (both in the general population and in the IVF population), there are far more chemical pregnancies diagnosed than clinical pregnancies in an IVF program.

As you would expect, statistics based on live births take into account the success rate based on the number of babies born from IVF cycles at the clinic. Live-birth rates are lower than both chemical and clinical pregnancy rates. A pregnancy rate based on either clinical or chemical pregnancies does tell you that the clinic is having some success, and it's for you to determine whether it's more important to know how many babies are actually born. It is worth considering the fact that, statistically, women who get pregnant (chemical or otherwise) and miscarry with IVF are more likely to go on and have a live birth than those who never get pregnant at all.

Another thing you need to consider when looking at success rates is the number of cycles performed by the clinic. As the guidelines to the CDC report point out, if a clinic only did one ART cycle, that clinic's success rate is going to be either 100 percent or 0 percent, depending on whether that patient got pregnant. Statistics from clinics that have high patient loads and do many cycles thus give you a more realistic picture of your chances than do success rates from clinics that do fewer cycles. If you need/want help understanding how to read the charts that clinics and the CDC use to publish success rates, I've placed a sample chart in the Appendix with a description of how to interpret the results.

So what's a good success rate? According to the American Society for Reproductive Medicine, the success rate for IVF nationally is around 20 percent. Don't let this number frighten you. This figure is low because it includes fertility centers with lousy statistics. There are many, many clinics that report success rates for women under thirty-five at around 50 percent per cycle (and some are even higher). If you are thirty-two years old with mild endometriosis, your chances of conceiving with IVF at a good clinic should be far greater than 20 percent. Be suspicious of anyone who claims a success rate over 65 percent. That's really hard to achieve, even at the best fertility centers in the world. Blastocyst transfer (discussed in chapter 12) success rates are slightly higher, but a success rate of more than 70 to 75 percent is suspiciously high. Blastocyst transfer success rates aren't officially reported (yet). If you're looking at a high number, check to see whether it refers to a chemical pregnancy rate, is limited to young patients (under thirty-two for example), or isn't audited or otherwise verified by an independent reviewer. Each of these factors can explain an unusually high success rate.

When comparing one clinic's success rate with another's, you also need to keep in mind that certain clinics have more liberal admission policies than others. Let's compare two hypothetical top-rated clinics. Both report success of rates of 50 percent for women under thirty-four. But Clinic A's success rates for women over forty are just 9 percent whereas Clinic B is reporting success rates of 39 percent. At first you think that Clinic B must be the better clinic because they have much better success rates for "older" women. You might even think that Clinic B is the right clinic for you because you're forty. Wrong! You need to know why Clinic A and Clinic B have such different success rates before you make your decision.

The truth is that some clinics are very fussy about who they let cycle, especially when it comes to women over forty. Nasty secret revealed: Clinic B won't treat many of the infertility patients in the over-forty category because it's just too hard to get them pregnant. Clinic B picks and chooses its over-forty patients and only cycles those women who have a good chance of conceiving. Clinic A, on the other hand, takes patients over forty (and even under forty) with certain very challenging infertility diagnoses and much lower chances of success.

Thus, if you are an average forty-year-old with a blocked fallopian tube (something that may be dealt with easily by IVF), Clinic A is just as good a place for you to cycle as Clinic B, even though Clinic A's success rates are drastically lower. Clinic B's success rates are much higher because the group of women they let cycle is more likely to get pregnant than those at Clinic A. If you don't have one of the conditions that would make it more difficult for you to conceive (high FSH for example, which we discuss in greater detail in the next chapter) and for which you're excluded from treatment at Clinic B, then Clinic A's lower success rate is *not* indicative of your chances of conceiving. In this case, you might want to find out what the success rate is at each clinic based on patients within your age group and with your diagnosis. Find out what each clinic's criteria are for treating patients and what types of diagnoses they will accept before you judge their success rates.

Finally, there are clinics of "last resort." It's horrible to refer to these clinics this way (I prefer to think of them as the "world-famous" clinics), but they're the ones that treat patients no one else can get pregnant. It is pretty amazing that these clinics—and there are really only a few of them worldwide—maintain the same success rates as other fertility centers but with a more challenging patient group. Usually, these clinics succeed because they have state-of-the-art facilities and some of the best reproductive physicians in the world, the ones who create new reproductive technologies. Your goal is to find a doctor who will give you the best chances of getting pregnant, right? Don't overlook the clinic of "last resort" because it seems too big, overwhelming, or expensive. If you have a complicated diagnosis or just want to increase your odds, you might do better starting off at one of these clinics.

After you've analyzed success rates and met with each doctor, give her a score based on your priorities and then write yourself a note that will remind you what most struck you about this doctor. When you have met with all the doctors on your list, you can sit down with your husband and your notes to decide who gets your business.

Let's say you've followed my advice to the letter and asked all the questions, and you can't decide which RE to pick. Consider the following:

- Do you have insurance that will pay for treatment?

- If so, how much coverage do you have? (See chapter 9.)

- Do any of the REs you've met with and like accept your insurance?

- If so, does the doctor that takes your insurance have lower success rates or inferior facilities to one of the doctors you met with who doesn't take your insurance?

- If you don't have insurance coverage or have limited coverage, how much can you afford to spend on infertility treatment?

- Do any of the programs offer financial assistance like shared-risk programs or low-interest private loans? (See chapter 9 for descriptions of these programs.)

- Is it worth going out of network at a more state-of-the-art facility if it means you will get pregnant faster? You might do just one cycle at the better center and pay $15,000 out of pocket, whereas you might do six cycles at the clinic that accepts your insurance before you get pregnant but not have to pay a penny.

- How patient a patient are you? What happens if you choose the clinic that doesn't accept insurance and you miscarry (oh, God, I hope not!) and have to try again?

Let's assume insurance isn't an issue for a moment:

- Do you have an RE locally that you like and that has good success rates and a good embryology lab?

- Do you have an RE locally that is okay, but there is someone at a bigger and better clinic that you like?

- How far do you have to travel to get treated at the bigger center?

- Can you commute daily?

- Can you afford to travel and stay in a hotel to get treated at the bigger clinic?

- Is the cost of traveling offset by the greater chance of succeeding on the first or second cycle at the bigger clinic?

- Can you take time off from work to travel to a distant clinic?

- Will it be more stressful to travel, or would it be better to be home with your family and your pets? (Believe it or not, some people find being away from home during an IVF cycle is less stressful.)

- If you have more than one good RE locally, which center or office is going to have a bigger wait in the morning for monitoring? (You can spend up to two hours in the morning getting blood work and ultrasounds done every day during your cycle.)

- Is a smaller office going to give you better, more personalized service?

Hopefully by answering these questions you have been able to narrow your choices somewhat. You may discover that you just can't afford not to try an IVF cycle or two with the doctor in your insurance plan, even though he doesn't have the greatest success rates. You may discover that being at the best possible facility is what you need and want.

Whatever you decide, remember not to be afraid of getting second or third opinions, especially when treatment isn't working for you. And if you need to, don't hesitate to switch doctors later in your treatment. Whatever else you do, promise me one thing: educate yourself *every step* of the way. (I talk about why I think this is so important in chapter 10.)

Now, let's find out exactly what's going on with you or your husband and what's preventing you from getting pregnant.

# 4

---

# Testing, Testing, Testing!

## FINDING OUT WHAT'S GOING ON AND
## WHAT'S GOING WRONG

Now that you have found a good RE, you're on your way to discovering what, if anything, is preventing you from getting pregnant. It's possible the first diagnostic test you'll have will reveal the culprit, and it's possible that you'll find out what's going wrong a year after your first test (remember, this is a *process*). But regardless of when and how you discover what's standing between you and a big fat beautiful stretch mark–covered belly, let me tell you about some of the tests you're likely to have and what they might tell you.

To make things simpler, I'm going to break each test down into sections describing "what it's for," "what's involved," and what to expect during "recovery." One last thing about this chapter (and others involving medical stuff): this stuff can be pretty dense to read. I have to put on my medical lab jacket and use my honorary M.D. (I got one from doing IVF so many times and having so many things wrong with me) to explain it. Please bear with me if it gets boring. The material is important, even if it's not that funny.

# Blood Tests

### SERUM PROGESTERONE BLOOD TEST

**What it's for:** Your RE may test your serum progesterone level to see if there is a problem with ovulation. Progesterone is a hormone that your body produces after ovulation to help support a pregnancy while the placenta is developing (it eventually will take over production of progesterone). This blood test is taken in the second half of your menstrual cycle, *after* you ovulate, to determine if your body is making progesterone; your RE wants to see a serum progesterone level above 12–15 ng/ml (nanograms per milliliter).

If your progesterone level is low, your doctor may suspect a luteal phase defect or other problem with ovulation. Together with other blood tests (FSH, LH, estradiol, and/or prolactin) and possibly an endometrial biopsy, your progesterone level will help give your RE a better sense of how well you're ovulating.

**What's involved:** A needle stick (for some of us this is a big deal) about a week after you ovulate.

**Recovery:** A Band-Aid, maybe.

### FSH, LH, AND ESTRADIOL BLOOD TESTS

**What it's for:** To evaluate your follicle stimulating hormone (FSH), luteinizing hormone (LH), and estradiol (E2) levels to determine the quality of your eggs.

Each RE and clinic will have different levels of FSH and LH that they deem acceptable. This is one test that's lab specific; if you interview multiple physicians, the test needs to be redone at the new physician's lab, as her lab may reach different values and ascribe different meanings to them (REs are trying to get a standard system of analyzing these levels, but they don't have it together yet). The general rule of thumb is that an

LH or FSH level greater than 13 mIU/ml (milli international units per milliliter) indicates there may be a problem with egg quality. An E2 level over 70 pg/ml (picograms per milliliter) may indicate an egg quality issue, too.

Your RE will also be looking at the relationship between your LH and FSH levels. A normal LH:FSH ratio shows the LH level lower than FSH. For example, a normal test might reveal a ratio of 5:11 (LH:FSH respectively). A higher LH than FSH level may indicate that you have polycystic ovarian syndrome (PCOS). An abnormally high FSH or E2 level may indicate premature ovarian failure. Women over forty tend to have higher FSH levels than thirty-year-old women (no one ever said the biological clock was fair). But different levels are not age-related. A young woman can have high FSH levels, and an older woman can have low FSH levels.

**What's involved:** A needle stick on the third day of your menstrual cycle.

**Recovery:** A Band-Aid, maybe.

### PROLACTIN AND ANDROGEN BLOOD TESTS

**What it's for:** High prolactin levels can interfere with ovulation; androgens are male hormones that also can interfere with ovulation. Prolactin and androgen levels help confirm diagnoses suspected from other test results. For example, if your doctor suspects you have PCOS, checking your androgen levels may help confirm her diagnosis, as higher than normal androgen levels are common among women with PCOS. If you've got irregular menstrual cycles, your RE may want to look at your prolactin level to see if that's interfering with your ovulation.

**What's involved:** A needle stick.

**Recovery:** Depending on how many blood tests you've had by now, a Band-Aid (and if you're anything like me, a super needle-phobe, a stiff drink).

## GENETIC TESTING FOR IVF FAILURE AND RECURRENT PREGNANCY LOSS

**What it's for:** Sometimes IVF cycles fail or women miscarry repeatedly due to a high number of chromosomally abnormal embryos. This is common in women over thirty-five and is even more common in women over forty, but it also happens with surprising frequency among all IVF patients. Recent research has identified a higher than expected incidence of chromosomally abnormal embryos produced during IVF procedures. The cause isn't yet known. Doctors are now encouraging patients who've had several IVF failures (in which you didn't get pregnant despite healthy looking embryos) or miscarriages to undergo genetic testing. This can be done in one of three ways, depending on the type of loss you're experiencing, and may help you identify treatments that could help you avoid another failure or loss.

**What's involved:** A genetic karyotyping is accomplished by a simple blood test and provides a complete analysis of your genetic makeup. Sometimes a gene is translocated (out of place), or there's something else in your genetic makeup that could lead to embryo death. If the test reveals something that could lead to miscarriage (or raise other problems later on in your baby's life), you can meet with a genetic counselor and discuss how you might be able to deal with the genetic issue.

For women experiencing miscarriages, there's a surgical procedure performed at the time of the miscarriage that can help determine whether your loss resulted from a chromosomal error. This procedure is called a D & C (dilation and curettage; I talk in more detail about the procedure in chapter 13), and it enables your RE to obtain tissue samples a pathologist can use to examine the genetic composition of the fetus. In medical terms it's called a cytogenic analysis. If the fetal tissue reveals a chromosomal error, you can have a karyotype analysis performed or talk to a genetic counselor.

It may also be worth considering using preimplantation genetic diagnosis (PGD, discussed in detail in chapter 7) if you've had several IVF failures or pregnancy losses. PGD examines the genetic composition of embryos and can help ensure that the embryos you transfer back to your uterus are genetically healthy. This can reduce your chances of experiencing another failure or loss.

**What's involved:** Genetic karyotyping involves a simple blood test. For women who've miscarried, the D & C surgery will retrieve fetal tissue for a genetic analysis (cytogenic report). For women contemplating an IVF cycle, you can talk to your RE about preimplantation genetic diagnosis. There are some risks (see chapter 7) involved in PGD, but beyond the "normal" experience of an IVF patient there isn't anything more involved for you. This testing is done on the embryo.

**Recovery:** For the blood test, nothing more than a Band-Aid. For a D & C, you will need to rest for a day or so after your surgical procedure. You may also have some bleeding and cramping for a few days.

## Immune Testing for IVF Failure and Recurrent Pregnancy Loss

**What it's for:** One of the newest areas of reproductive medicine is based on reproductive immunology. Your immune system, which protects you from colds and flu bugs, might also play a role in your IVF or pregnancy failure. Most immune testing is done on women—like me—who suffer from recurrent pregnancy loss (which is exactly what it sounds like, recurrent miscarriage) and IVF failure (when you fail to get pregnant with IVF despite numerous attempts and healthy embryos). Some reproductive centers include immune testing as part of their initial workup. Most centers, however, haven't yet accepted this field of reproductive medicine—it's quite controversial; many REs think this stuff is bunk—so if you think you might benefit from testing, you may have to fight for it. The testing involves fairly specialized and expensive (more than $2,000, which is often not covered by insurance) blood work to see if you have antibodies or blood-clotting issues that could prevent you from achieving or maintaining a pregnancy. Most of the time, a daily baby aspirin and prescription vitamins with high-dose folic acid, $B_6$, and $B_{12}$ can solve the problem. Some women may need a prescription blood thinner in addition to baby aspirin and/or vitamin supplementation.

If you're only able to allocate one attempt at IVF, then consider getting these tests done as a precaution, even if you have to find another doctor to do the immune workup. It would be horrible to find out after stopping IVF that baby aspirin and a prescription vitamin or even one shot a day of a prescription blood thinner might've made the difference between failure and success. If you think you might benefit from testing but can't find anyone to run the tests for you, I've listed some of the physicians who deal with this stuff in the Resources section.

There are three categories of immune issues that can affect pregnancy. They are: blood-clotting disorders, problems with certain antibodies, and baby-killing cells. These labels obviously aren't the terms used by reproductive immunologists (and will probably raise a few eyebrows among medical professionals). But there's so much overlap between the names and types of problems that your head would start spinning if I tried to explain it in any greater detail. If you get a diagnosis for one of these conditions, you can read about treatment for it in chapter 5.

## TESTS FOR BLOOD-CLOTTING DISORDERS

**What it's for:** Normally, a woman's ability to make blood clots in the uterine environment is suppressed during a pregnancy. This ensures that blood flows to the growing fetus, and that the blood flow will increase as the baby gets bigger. If you have a thrombophiliac condition—a blood-clotting disorder—clots can form that restrict the flow of blood to the baby. This can happen at the site of implantation, in the placenta, or in veins and arteries that support the pregnancy and can prevent implantation, cause early pregnancy loss and intrauterine growth retardation (where the baby's growth is inhibited), among other problems (yes, there are more).

There are two types of thrombophilias (blood-clotting disorders): those that are inherited from your parents and those that you acquire during your lifetime. The inherited thrombophilias generally result from a genetic mutation or abnormal levels of certain proteins essential to maintaining normal clotting functions. These blood-clotting disorders include (but aren't limited to), Leiden factor V mutation R560Q, mutations to the MTHFR gene (trust me, you don't want me to spell out the full name, it's a tongue twister if ever there was one!), prothrombin gene mutation 20210 (GA), and abnormal protein C or protein S levels.

Certain gene mutations, like the double recessive (homozygous) mutation of MTHFR, can cause other long-term health problems. If you're diagnosed with a blood-clotting disorder due to one of these conditions, you may need to have regular blood monitoring (ask your doctor about it); the homozygous mutation (double recessive) of the MTHFR gene (what I have) places me at high risk for developing a condition known as hyperhomocysteinemia. Hyperhomocysteinemia is thought to play a role in the development of heart disease and Alzheimer's. Because I have this mutation, I will pass the defect on to any biological children I may have.

**What's involved:** An expensive blood test (about $1,000).

**Recovery:** A Band-Aid.

### TESTS FOR ANTIBODY PROBLEMS

**What it's for:** Certain types of antibodies may also cause blood-clotting problems and other autoimmune issues. These are the acquired (as opposed to inherited) thrombophilias I mentioned earlier. There are four different categories of antibodies to look for: antiphospholipid antibodies (APA), antithyroid antibodies, antinuclear antibodies (ANA), and lupuslike anticoagulant antibodies. Research suggests that up to 30 percent of women suffering from recurrent miscarriage will show abnormalities with one or more of these antibodies. Let's talk about the antiphospholipid antibodies (APA) first.

Your doctor has probably already tested you for one kind of phospholipids (anticardiolipins) but in order to really diagnose a problem with APA, you must look for the presence of six additional antibodies. (Trust me, you don't really need to know the names of each antibody; suffice it to say they belong to the Igm, IgG, and IgA classes, and even this isn't really necessary to know, I'm just showing off my honorary M.D. again!) Testing positive for one or more of these antibodies is an indication you're having or are at risk for an autoimmune response that causes (among other things) implantation failure and miscarriage.

A small subset of women with recurrent pregnancy loss test positive for lupuslike anticoagulant antibodies (and no, you don't have lupus if you test positive). Your doctor can perform an easy screen to see if you might be in this group by performing a standard test on your blood clotting time, known as the activated partial thromboplastin time (APTT). If these results are abnormal, more sensitive testing should be done to determine the presence of lupus anticoagulant antibodies.

The third type of antibody you should be screened for are antinuclear antibodies (ANA). ANA can be present in other immunologic diseases like lupus (again, testing positive for ANA doesn't mean you have lupus), or in people with certain vascular diseases. Testing positive for ANA indicates some sort of autoimmune response to the development of the placenta; it isn't clear how this causes pregnancy loss. One little quirk about ANA is that it's possible to test in the normal range for ANA when you're not pregnant and test in the abnormal range when you are. Repeat testing during pregnancy is recommended.

The fourth category of antibodies is called antithyroid antibodies. There are two types of antithyroid antibodies, thyroglobulin and thyroid peroxidase. Elevated levels of these antibodies are thought to double your risk of miscarriage. It is believed that as many as 31 percent of women who suffer from recurrent pregnancy loss test positive for one of these two antibodies. If you have any kind of thyroid disorder, you should have these antibodies tested.

The live birth rate among women treated for these conditions (usually treatment is with baby aspirin or heparin) is around 70 percent. Multiple miscarriage before treatment reduces the chances of success, especially if you've had more than five losses. If you're pregnant and have a history of recurrent pregnancy loss, it's not too late to get tested. Repeat and initial testing during pregnancy is recommended for patients with prior loss and/or a positive antibody test.

**What's involved:** An expensive blood test ($1,000–$2,000, could be over $2,000 if done by a reproductive immunologist).

**Recovery:** A Band-Aid (and maybe a Kamikaze shot when you're paying your Visa bill).

### TESTS FOR BABY-KILLING CELLS

**What it's for:** Every body has immune cells that seek out and destroy foreign invaders. In a normal pregnancy, the mother's immune system recognizes the father's genetic material (human leukocyte antigens or HLA) as different from the mother's and creates antibodies that protect the fetus from these destroyer cells. If, however, the father's genetic material (his HLA) is too similar to that of the mother's, her body won't make the protective antibodies. Her body's destroyer cells then attack the developing fetus. HLA tissue typing (done through blood tests) can help identify couples that may have this problem and are at risk for miscarriage.

Two other types of problems with baby-killing cells arise when your body makes too many natural killer and other cells that are toxic to embryos (embryotoxic cells). Natural killer cells (known as NK cells) seek out and destroy things like cancer cells by secreting something known as tumor necrosis factor or TNF. TNF is toxic to embryos. Patients with high levels of certain NK cells in the uterine environment also have high levels of TNF, which can increase their risk of miscarriage. A reproductive immunophenotype test (RIP test) looks for these types of NK cells and can identify high-risk patients.

The embryotoxic cells are called cytokines. Some stimulate cell growth, while others prevent growth by causing an inflammatory response in the body. An embryo toxicity assay (ETA) looks for cytokines that cause inflammation that can lead to embryo death. Abnormal levels of cytokines are not uncommon in women with endometriosis.

**What's involved:** Blood tests can look for all of these abnormal cell conditions. More sophisticated testing of uterine tissue (removed during a D & C) can also be performed to identify the presence of these antibodies and killer cells. If you haven't had a D & C after a miscarriage, you'll have to start with blood tests. If you've already had a D & C, your hospital should have saved tissue samples that can be sent to a reproductive immunologist for further testing (not always necessary for diagnosis, but superaggressive women, like me, may choose to do this). Check out the Resources section for names of doctors to do this testing. Blood testing can cost about $1,000; the D & C and pathology review of tissue can cost several thousand dollars but should be covered by most insurance.

**Recovery:** Depends on whether you had the blood work or a D & C. It's anything from a boo-boo bandage to a couple of days in bed. You're probably getting over the sticker shock by now.

## More Invasive Tests

In addition to blood tests, your RE may want to take a sample of your endometrial lining and/or examine the inside of your uterine cavity and fallopian tubes. The upside is that this testing is relatively simple to perform—in fact, it usually can be done during your lunch hour—and can tell your doctor *a lot* about what is going on with your reproductive system. The downside is that it can be uncomfortable (okay, if I'm going to be honest, some of them are downright *painful*).

## ENDOMETRIAL BIOPSY

**What it's for:** This helps your doctor determine whether your uterine lining and hormonal system are sufficiently in sync to sustain a pregnancy.

Before ovulation, your uterine lining (your endometrium) should thicken and develop blood vessels that will help nourish and support an embryo. If the development of your uterine lining is not precisely timed with ovulation, you may not achieve successful implantation (a pregnancy), even though you fertilized an egg. This condition is known as a luteal phase defect (or LPD). Although your blood tests may indicate you had a normal ovulation, you may need a biopsy to confirm that your uterus is ready to receive and nurture a fertilized egg. For example, if your luteal phase (the time between when you ovulate and get your period) is less than twelve days, you likely have LPD, and your doctor may want to confirm that diagnosis with a biopsy of your uterine lining. Only a pathologist's analysis of cells from your uterine lining can reveal the developmental stage of the lining.

**What's involved:** The biopsy is generally performed eleven to thirteen days after the surge of hormones (LH) that immediately precedes ovulation, or one to three days before your next period. It's not a big deal; it can be performed in your RE's office and doesn't take very long.

It will seem like a regular GYN exam at first, stirrups, speculum, vulnerability, embarrassment, and all the usual dreaded GYN exam stuff. After the speculum (which hopefully your RE is evolved enough to know should be *warmed up* before insertion), she will insert a small catheter through the opening in your cervix (the cervical os). The catheter may pinch a little, but you probably won't feel it at all. Next, using a syringe attached to the end of the catheter, your RE essentially will suck a piece of endometrial tissue from your uterus (another technique involves taking a scraping of a piece of uterine lining). You may feel a slight tugging sensation or a sharp cramp as the tissue is removed. It can be painful. (I've had two performed; one didn't hurt at all and one hurt like hell; go figure!) The process of removing the tissue only takes about a minute.

**A word to the wise:** | One thing you may want to try drilling into your partner's thick skull early on in this process is that the amount of crap you're going to go through to have this baby far exceeds the small— shall we say *minute*—inconveniences that (s)he has to endure (which we shall discuss later in this book). Thus, your significant other should respond to every procedure, injection, and exam with flowers, cards, presents, take-out food, or whatever it is that makes you happy. It may sound pathetic, but knowing that I'm going to get a little TLC on the day of a procedure makes it a little easier to bear.

From start (speculum insertion) to finish (speculum removal), the whole procedure should take five to ten minutes.

If you are truly a chicken—like me—you can ask your RE for a small dose of a mood relaxing drug before the procedure. You also may be able to take a pain reliever before the biopsy to help minimize the cramping. Your RE may prefer that you take a low dose narcotic or extra strength acetaminophen rather than a nonsteroidal anti-inflammatory drug like Aleve or Motrin (these can cause additional bleeding), so ask your physician what she recommends.

**Recovery:** Slight cramping and bleeding or spotting after the procedure is completely normal. An endometrial biopsy can be performed on your lunch hour, but if you're anything like me, once the procedure is done, you will want to go home where, after congratulating yourself on being such a trooper, you can change into comfy clothes, curl up on the couch, and watch Oprah while enjoying a glass of wine (skip the wine if you took any kind of medication to get through the procedure). This, too, is a good time to demand take-out Chinese for dinner and a little pampering from your husband.

A few last comments about endometrial biopsies: first, they really are worth doing. Many women try to avoid them because of the potential pain factor, but they're truly useful in helping to identify impediments to pregnancy. Second, you shouldn't try to conceive in the cycle when you have it done; taking a piece of lining away from an embryo is *not* a good idea and can result in an early miscarriage. And third, if you're really afraid of pain (who isn't?) and your RE is discussing performing a laparoscopy or hysteroscopy (we'll talk about these in a minute), ask her if she'll do the biopsy during the surgery when you're anesthetized. I hate to say it, but doing them separately means she can bill you separately, so she might prefer to do the biopsy first and the surgery second. If you want them done together, ask her to do them together. She'll probably comply. Might as well multitask while you're out for the count!

## HYSTEROSALPINOGRAM (HSG)

**What it's for:** This may be one of the most useful nonsurgical diagnostic tools in your RE's arsenal. It is a sophisticated X ray that allows your RE to look inside your uterine cavity and fallopian tubes to determine if both are structurally normal.

**What's involved:** The HSG—don't even try to pronounce the full name of this test; everyone calls it an HSG, except your RE (and she's just showing off)—takes about a half hour and is performed at the hospital usually in the beginning or middle of your menstrual cycle, before ovulation. You will be given antibiotics to take for a few days after the procedure to prevent infection. This can be a very uncomfortable test, but there is little way of predicting whether yours will be painless or not.

It works like this: You get on top of a large table underneath an X-ray machine, and you put your feet in stirrups. Your doctor inserts a speculum (at this point in your testing you almost don't notice this part) and then a catheter through your cervix into your uterine cavity. Through the catheter, your RE will inject a dye (or contrast solution) that is visible (it's white) on the X-ray machine. This allows your RE to see the shape of your uterine cavity and any abnormalities (polyps or fibroids) and whether the dye flows through your fallopian tubes. If it doesn't flow through, your tubes are probably obstructed (this may well be why you're not getting pregnant).

The HSG is often most painful if there are uterine abnormalities or tubal obstructions. If, for example, the dye is unable to flow out one of your fallopian tubes because it's blocked, the pressure can be painful (believe me, I know). When everything is normal, women report that this test is completely painless. The skill of the physician performing the HSG also factors into the pain scale.

Diagnosing a problem within the fallopian tube is most often achieved by HSG. The good news about having an HSG is that the procedure itself often resolves tubal blockages and obstructions.

If your doctor sees an obstruction during your HSG, she can peform a tubal catheterization (also called a transcervical cannulation). Using small guide wires, catheters are inserted in your uterus and then moved up into the fallopian tube. Fluid is then flushed through the catheters in an effort to push the blockage out. This procedure effectively reopens blocked tubes about 50 percent of the time. Surgery may be needed to repair more severe blockages. A laparoscopy may later be performed to assess the nature and severity of the blockage and attempt to fix it.

If you're at an infertility clinic and the doctors rotate doing HSGs, you might want to ask around about which physician (sometimes it's a radiologist) is the gentlest, and schedule your HSG for a day that doctor is on duty. One of my friends was able to find out which of the REs at her clinic had the happiest post-HSG patients and asked for that doctor to perform her HSG. She found the HSG to be mildly uncomfortable but hardly painful. And the other day I heard about a woman whose HSG was completely painless (lucky woman!).

The good news about HSGs is that many women get pregnant shortly after having one. The theory is that the dye flushes all your reproductive plumbing clean (or as in my case, resolves an obstruction) thus facilitating a pregnancy. Many REs recommend having an HSG done before you begin to take any kind of medication like Clomid to help you ovulate. If there is an obstruction in one or both of your fallopian tubes, there is no point taking medication to help you ovulate if the sperm and egg can't meet in the fallopian tube or if there is another abnormality that would prevent implantation. If the dye flushes everything clean and you take Clomid the following month, you'll have a better chance of conceiving. In fact, this happened to my sister-in-law; after three years of trying to conceive, she got pregnant the month after her HSG. It might hurt like a bitch, but it's worthwhile.

**Recovery:** You may have some minor cramping after the procedure or feel bruised (I felt bloated and bruised). Take acetaminophen or something like Aleve, grab a heating pad, have a glass of wine, rent a good chick flick, put your legs up, and watch your partner fold the laundry (for a change).

## SALINE SONOGRAM OR SALINE HSG

**What it's for:** This test is a lot easier to tolerate than HSGs, and it's pretty effective at revealing what may be going on (or wrong) in your uterine cavity (it's far less helpful at identifying problems with your fallopian tubes).

**What's involved:** During this test your doctor will insert a speculum and then pushes a small catheter through your cervix into your uterine cavity. The catheter is attached to a syringe filled with saline solution that will be injected into your uterus. This is fairly painless. You may feel some cramping as the catheter goes in or as your uterus fills with the fluid. It's nothing compared even to a mild menstrual cramp and isn't something to worry about.

After the catheter has been inserted into your uterine cavity, the doctor will remove the speculum (but not the catheter) and insert an ultrasound transducer (I fondly refer to this device as the Magic Love Wand as it vaguely resembles a sex toy). An ultrasound monitor will then display a small oval blob on its screen, your uterus. Next, your RE injects the saline solution through the catheter. The uterine lining, your endometrium, moves aside as the saline enters the cavity, and your doctor can then see what, if anything, is embedded in or attached to your uterine lining.

When I had mine done, Dr. Chung saw a small polyp in my uterus. I thought it looked like a chili pepper hanging from the side of my uterus. I had some mild—not too horrible—cramping. What really bothered me was the gush of fluid out my whazoo and onto the floor when I stood up. No one warned me about this! I highly recommend holding an absorbent pad between your legs when you stand (take the one they put under your tush before the procedure). This way you will avoid making a puddle on the floor between your feet (very embarrassing, even if it's happened to dozens of women).

**Recovery:** You really won't need any painkillers after a saline HSG, but don't tell that to your significant other. Milk it for all it's worth. Maybe he should cook you dinner for once!

Now comes the more invasive surgical procedures. Your doctor may want to perform one or more of these to help confirm a suspected diagnosis (like endometriosis) or to remove a growth she discovered during your HSG (like a fibroid or polyp in your uterine cavity).

### HYSTEROSCOPY

**What it's for:** A hysteroscopy is often performed when your RE knows there's a problem, like a uterine polyp or fibroid diagnosed during your HSG, and wants to take a closer look so she can remove whatever s/he finds. The advantage of this procedure (other than the fact you're anesthetized) is that your doctor can correct an impediment to pregnancy without making a surgical cut in your abdomen or uterine wall. The disadvantage is that any problems with your ovaries (adhesions or scarring from infection or endometriosis) cannot be corrected or even visualized. This is because your doctor does not perform the hysteroscopy through an incision in your abdomen. She's going to go in through your cervix and looks only at your uterus.

**What's involved:** The hysteroscopy is the least invasive of the reproductive surgical procedures. While you're anesthetized for the procedure and will need to rest for a day or so afterward, the recovery time and discomfort level you may experience afterward are much less intense than with a laparoscopy (discussed next).

Your RE will insert a small telescopic device with an attached fiber optic light through your cervix and into your uterus. A small amount of liquid or carbon dioxide gas, released through the scope into your uterine cavity, expands it so that your doctor can see inside your uterus and can repair or remove any problem-causing abnormalities.

**Recovery:** There is very little discomfort after this procedure. You'll probably only experience some mild cramping and spotting. You may be very tired from the anesthesia. You will go home from the hospital the same day and should be pampered by your mate. Watch a good video, read a good book, or just sleep.

One important note: the hysteroscopy can be (and often is) performed in conjunction with a laparoscopy. When performed together, these procedures enable your RE to see (and repair) all your reproductive organs at the same time. If your RE is discussing performing a laparoscopy, you might want to ask whether she'll consider or is planning on performing a hysteroscopy. Multitask!

## LAPAROSCOPY

**What it's for:** A laparoscopy is a surgical procedure used to diagnose and correct certain fertility problems like endometriosis.

**What's involved:** This surgery requires two or three (sometimes more) small incisions in your abdomen. Through these incisions—generally made in your belly button and on each side of your lower abdomen (so small you won't have scars!)—your RE inserts a telescopic device with a fiber optic light, a laparoscope, and injects carbon dioxide gas to your abdominal cavity. The gas expands your belly and pushes organs out of the way so your doctor can clearly see the outside of your uterus, ovaries, and intestines.

Your doctor will be able to see any adhesions (scar tissue) or other abnormalities from endometriosis or infections. Your fallopian tubes will probably be flushed with fluid (called hydrotubation, for the medically oriented) to make sure they're open, the surface of your ovaries will be examined in detail (your RE can tell if you've been ovulating depending on the smoothness of the surface of your ovary), the fimbria or hair at the end of your fallopian tubes (the things that grab the egg when it's released from the ovary at ovulation) will be examined, the inside and outside of your uterus may be looked at, your cervix, and even your bowel; you name it and it gets scrutinized and photographed. The next question is whether you really want to see these pictures; your doctor may want to show them to you.

Any abnormalities—adhesions, cysts, fibroids, endometriosis lesions—can be surgically corrected either with a laser (to burn tissue away) or other small instruments inserted through the laparoscope. Once the procedure is completed, your little incisions (they tend to look like puncture wounds) are stitched up and an adhesive bandage is placed over them.

**Recovery:** After the anesthesia wears off you will be fairly uncomfortable but you will get to go home. At first the most painful part of the laparoscopy is the gas pain—sometimes you feel it up by your shoulders. Your lower abdomen will be extremely bloated (I thought I looked about six months' pregnant) and it will be *very* tender. Depending on how much corrective work your doctor does, you may need several days in bed (or on the couch) to recover.

I have had two laparoscopies (a year apart) and both times I was diagnosed with fairly severe endometriosis. My doctor was able to clean most of it up each time. Unfortunately, all that cleaning up meant I had what felt like major surgery (albeit outpatient) and wasn't able to get in and out of bed easily for several days. Percocet was my best friend. However, I have friends who were back at work in two or three days after laparoscopies. Because recovery times can vary dramatically from patient to patient, you should talk to your RE about how long your recovery is expected to take.

# Getting Your Diagnosis

WHAT'S WRONG WITH ME?

You may have a bunch of scary names whirling around your head right now. Take a deep breath. You're going to be okay. I promise!

Some of this discussion is a little detailed and even dry. I want you to understand as much as possible about your condition so you can make intelligent choices about treating it. So forgive me while I don the white lab coat again. (I promise at some point I'll throw it in the trash!) Just in case you don't want to read every detail about the diagnoses discussed, I've broken everything down into two sections: one describes the condition ("What it is") and the other how to treat it ("Treatment").

## Endometriosis

**What it is:** Endometriosis is believed to be a genetic disorder of the immune system that affects the reproductive system. Endometriosis is caused (at least in part) by retrograde menstruation, or backflow of menstrual blood and tissue through the fallopian tubes and into the abdominal cavity, where it causes scarring and adhesions. All women experience retrograde menstruation to some degree, so it's unclear why and how this tissue grows outside the uterine cavity and causes problems for some women and not others. Nor is it clear why some women have severe cases and others don't, or why some women with the disease have infertility problems and/or suffer miscarriages and others don't. There is, however, a clear link between the severity of the disease and infertility. Doctors know one thing for certain: the more severe your endometriosis is, the more difficult it may be for you to conceive.

While endo is a poorly understood disease, and its genetic origins are only now being researched, doctors have established that patients whose sister(s) or mother have endometriosis are 60 percent (or greater) more likely to have it than those whose relatives don't have it. There's a huge international gene study under way to find whether endometriosis is genetic and to identify the gene. Check out the Resources section at the back of the book if you want to learn more about the study and, perhaps, participate. I believe in the genetic link as my mother, her twin, and one of their sisters all had surgically diagnosed endometriosis.

Doctors know that endometriosis is painful and impairs fertility in up to 40 percent of patients who have it; current estimates are that as many as five million women suffer from endometriosis.

Endo (as it's fondly known by those of us who suffer from it) can be found on your bowel, your bladder, and inside your fallopian tubes, just to name a few places. It has been discovered all over the body, including places not even remotely positioned near reproductive organs (yuck!). When the disease is active, the tissue grows outside the uterus, stimulated by the same hormones that cause it to grow inside the uterus. The tissue eventually dies and causes scar tissue or adhesions; sadly, dead tissue doesn't mean dead disease. New tissue continues to grow and spread and causes pain and a greater potential for infertility. The longer endo goes untreated, the more likely you are to become infertile. Women with the disease usually have obstructed fallopian tubes and/or damaged ovaries (not to mention fibroids and polyps) among many other problems that can interfere with fertility.

Endometriosis is usually associated with very painful menstrual periods. We're talking take a day off from work and throw up kind of pain (some lucky women experience milder forms of discomfort). Symptoms also can include heavy flow during your period, pain at or during ovulation (sometimes severe), irritable bowel syndrome–like symptoms (constipation, diarrhea, and/or severe bowel cramping), pain during intercourse, and bloating. You can have one of the symptoms or all of them. It's rare, but it's possible to have endometriosis without any outward symptoms. The bottom line—as I have learned—is that pain with menses is not normal (can you believe you were *taught* it is normal?), and any regular (as in every month) and uncomfortable menstrual cramping should be mentioned to your doctor. It is *not* in your head!

Endometriosis is often discovered after symptoms appear (heavy and painful periods) or after an ultrasound or pelvic exam. Another hallmark of the disease is hemorrhagic cysts (called endometriomas) on the ovary. An endometrioma, or "chocolate cyst," is a cyst on the ovary filled with blood that thickens over time, turns to a chocolaty-like substance, and oozes from the cyst when it is drained (as a chocolate lover, this kind of grosses me out!). I get them all the time; and by the way, they can hurt. Endo cannot officially be diagnosed without surgery (usually a laparoscopy) and a subsequent examination of tissue.

Endo can interfere with fertility in several ways. It can cause scarring in the fallopian tubes that makes them impassable to sperm and egg. And it can cause structural abnormalities on the ovary or in the uterus that interfere with ovulation or implantation. Doctors also suspect that women with endo have some idiosyncrasy in their immune system that makes them more likely to miscarry.

**Treatment:** The more advanced your endo is, the more scarring and adhesions you have. Stage I (minimal endo) or stage II (mild endo) may not impact on your fertility at all; stage III (moderate endo) and stage IV endo can make life extremely challenging in terms of both day-to-day life and in getting pregnant. The good news is that even severe, stage IV endo (like I have) can be treated with surgery and medication and doesn't mean you won't get pregnant. I have several friends with advanced, stage III or stage IV, endo and they all have IVF babies.

If you or your doctor suspects you have endo, I suggest you schedule a laparoscopy as soon as possible. Some doctors prefer to wait and see if the symptoms subside or disappear (hoping you don't really have endo) as the surgery is kind of a big deal. However, if you've got a family history of endo or long-term symptoms, then having the surgery sooner rather than later may improve your chances of conceiving. The laparoscopy can clean your organs up (bowel, bladder, and ovaries included), which should reduce your pain and prepare you for infertility treatments like IVF, which is the treatment of choice for women with moderate to severe endometriosis, because it completely bypasses the fallopian tubes and helps ensure a healthy ovulation, two problems/impediments that are common among women with endo. (See Chapter 7 for more information on IVF.)

You can also choose to take medication that shuts down your reproductive system (yes, that means no attempts at conception), like birth control pills or Lupron and Synarel (you can read more about these meds in chapter 11, although the dosage differs from that given to IVF patients). Without hormonal support and the retrograde flow of menstrual blood, endometrial tissue stops migrating and growing. Essentially, you kill the disease for the period of time you're on the medication. Taking medication before surgery can make surgical repairs easier for your RE; taking medication after surgery may extend the period of time you've got before symptoms return. Once you go off the medication, your endo will come back. Together or separately, these treatments can effectively lessen your pain and restore or improve your fertility.

If you do have a laparoscopy, please keep in mind that the best time to conceive a baby is the six months to one year following your surgery. After those six months—depending on the severity of your endo—you may need to consider more surgery or consider alternative family building options (see chapter 7). Keep in mind, too, that for some women the drugs used during IUI and IVF cycles can increase the rate of advancement of the disease. (Remember when I said there were many double-edged swords in infertility treatment land? This is one of them!) When you've been diagnosed with endo, you want to be aggressive and decisive about infertility treatment. You may have a very limited window in which to work before you need more surgery.

Other effective ways to treat endo include dietary changes and acupuncture. After my second laparoscopy, I was determined not to have a third. I read up on the connection between diet and the immune system and about the success many women had in restoring endo-impaired fertility by changing their diet and using acupuncture. (If you're into it, check out the Resources section for the book I read that helped me make these changes.) Making significant—but not restrictive—dietary changes vastly reduced the rate of development of my disease. Four months after I changed my diet, my periods became a lot less painful and heavy. I haven't needed a laparoscopy since then, and I am almost four years past my last surgery (the first two were barely a year apart). Dietary changes can be used to treat fibroids as well.

## Fallopian Tubes and Other Structural Problems

**What it is:** The fallopian tubes are necessary for natural conception but are unnecessary for getting pregnant with IVF. In a natural pregnancy, the fallopian tube is the conduit between the egg and sperm (the egg travels down the fallopian tube, and the sperm travels up the tube to meet the egg). Fertilization takes place in the tube, and the embryo first begins to grow and obtain life-supporting nutrients there as well. Accordingly, if there is a blockage or narrowing of some portion of the tube, the egg and sperm may not be able to reach each other. If the mucosal lining of the tube has been damaged, a fertilized egg may not be able to get the nutrients it needs to survive (as the fertilized egg rolls and bumps its way down the fallopian tube, it gets nourishment from substances that exist in the mucous lining of the tube). The fallopian tube can be damaged by endometriosis, infection, pelvic inflammatory disease (PID), or prior pelvic or abdominal surgery. Also, a prior ruptured appendix in childhood or adolescence notoriously causes scarring in the right fallopian tube. Diseased or damaged fallopian tubes account for about 20 to 30 percent of all causes of infertility.

**Treatment:** Microsurgery is the best way to repair a damaged fallopian tube. However, it may not be your best bet for getting pregnant.

Tubal microsurgery may be performed during a laparoscopy to repair fallopian tube damage that has been detected during a previous HSG or during the laparoscopy itself. Microsurgery is often successful, but more complicated corrective procedures don't always offer great results, even when performed by a very skilled surgeon. Unfortunately, many times the microsurgery to repair a damaged tube often doesn't restore your ability to conceive a baby the old-fashioned way (sex). Success rates—the likelihood that a couple will conceive the old-fashioned way after surgery—vary dramatically, depending on the skill of the surgeon performing the procedure and the complexity or type of surgical repair you require.

I'm going to give you for success rates for various types of tubal microsurgeries. Don't freak when you read these numbers; having your fallopian tubes surgically repaired isn't your only path to pregnancy. IVF is a *great* option for conceiving when you have diseased or damaged fallopian tubes, and means you can choose to bypass this surgery altogether if you want to. But if you're inclined to try the surgical repair route, take the time to find a really skilled surgeon (contact the American Society for Reproductive Medicine for a good referral); your chances of conceiving may be pretty decent. Your prospect may be even better than my statistics suggest because the medical techniques and procedures are always improving, and the most recent statistics available are a few years old.

Surgery to repair fallopian tubes substantially increases the risk of ectopic pregnancy, which occurs within the fallopian tube and isn't viable, and can jeopardize your life. In the normal population the risk of an ectopic pregnancy is about .5 percent. The risk of ectopic pregnancy after tubal repair is significant.

- If your fallopian tube has to be *resected* (meaning a portion of it is cut out and the two ends are surgically reattached; it's called rean-astomosed for those interested in medical terms), success rates run about 50 percent (meaning 50 percent of patients having the surgery will achieve a pregnancy afterward) with a risk of conceiving an ectopic pregnancy approaching 10 percent.

- The correction of a *hydrosalpinx*, a closure of the fallopian tube near the top by your ovary, which results in a fluid-filled sac (think of it like a tiny balloon created by your fallopian tube), results in a 25 percent chance of conceiving but with a much higher risk of de-veloping an ectopic pregnancy, somewhere between 20 and 50 per-cent.

- *Closures at both ends of the tube* are perhaps the most difficult to repair surgically and have the lowest success rate, only a 5 percent chance of conceiving a baby the old-fashioned way after surgery.

- *If your fallopian tubes were tied* as a method of permanent birth con-trol (tubal ligation), the tubes can be untied surgically, often restor-ing fertility. Success rates for the repair of a tubal ligation run as high as 80 percent.

If you're considering surgery to correct tubal infertility, you should first speak with your doctor about your ovarian reserve (discussed later in this chapter), sperm quality, and the overall health of your reproductive system. You will have a better chance at conception after surgery if both partners' reproductive systems work optimally. Know, too, that tubal sur-geries can only be performed once; the success rate for multiple tubal microsurgical procedures is pretty dismal.

So, while microsurgery can resolve tubal infertility, you should weigh the risks and benefits of these procedures against the fact that IVF elim-inates the need for the fallopian tube altogether. Your best and fastest bet to achieving a pregnancy might be to proceed straight to IVF. I discuss this option in chapter 7.

## Fibroids and Polyps

**What it is:** I lump these two conditions together because they are similar. Both are growths usually found within the uterine cavity, and can—but don't always—interfere with fertility. The treatment—surgery—is similar, too, but the type of surgical procedure differs depending on whether you've got fibroids or polyps.

Approximately 25 percent of women have fibroids during their reproductive lifetime. These are noncancerous growths or tumors in the wall of the uterine muscle. You generally don't just have one fibroid; most women have several (as many as seven at a time). They can grow within the muscle wall, protrude into the uterine cavity, or grow outside of the uterus. Interestingly, African American women are up to five times more likely to develop fibroids than Caucasian women. This supports a genetic predisposition to the development of fibroids and, in fact, researchers at the Center for Uterine Fibroids at Brigham and Women's Hospital in Boston, Massachusetts, have identified mutations in two genes that appear to be related to the development of fibroids. (For more information on the Center for Uterine Fibroids, see the Resources section; they have a gene study under way, if you're interested in participating.) Fibroids are also more common in women who are overweight, smoke, and who've given birth.

The most common symptom of fibroids is abnormal or heavy uterine bleeding. If your periods last more than four days or are so heavy that you change your maxi pad every hour (gross!) or restrict your activities to avoid an embarrassing accident (ugh!), you might want to check with your doctor to see if you have a fibroid(s). You might also feel bloated (especially if the fibroid is so large that your uterus has grown and is pressing on your bladder or bowel) or experience excessive menstrual cramping. Fibroids are often discovered during a routine pelvic exam but can also be detected with an ultrasound, MRI, HSG, saline HSG, hysteroscopy, or laparoscopy.

Though otherwise benign, fibroids can interfere with conception and the development of a pregnancy. Large fibroids that distort the shape of the uterus or are located toward the top of the uterine cavity—where most embryos make their home—can prevent an embryo from successfully implanting. Other fibroids can interfere with blood supply to the embryo (as some fibroids need blood to survive and essentially tap into blood vessels and veins that might otherwise nourish a developing fetus) or get in the way of a growing fetus (sometimes this isn't problematic to the fetus but is painful for the mother). Fibroids on the external wall aren't going to impact your chances of conceiving but will need to be monitored for growth and interruption of the function of other organs (like your bladder).

Polyps, like fibroids, are benign growths that don't always interfere with implantation and pregnancy. Unlike fibroids, polyps aren't likely to pose a problem once you're pregnant. Compared to fibroids, polyps are soft and squish out of the way of a growing baby. They are more common among women in their fifties than women of childbearing age, but believe me (as I've had them), they can pop up in your early thirties. The most common symptom of polyps is bleeding between periods or excessive spotting after your period. Polyps generally cannot be felt during a pelvic exam (they're so soft they squish out of the way), but they can be seen on ultrasound or during an HSG.

**Treatment:** If your RE isn't concerned about them playing a role in pregnancy achievement, you can leave polyps alone. But if they interfere or the bleeding is bothering you, you might want to get rid of them. Most likely, your doctor will suggest that you have a hysteroscopy (remember, this way she can see everything in the uterine cavity so she knows she cleans everything up) so she can remove the polyp(s).

The most common treatment for *fibroids* is a hysterectomy. This "cures" the problem altogether. However, for those of us who want to preserve our fertility and are in fact trying to get pregnant, there are other options. If your doctor recommends a hysterectomy for fibroids and you're trying to have a baby, *find another doctor*. Skillful, trained surgeons can perform a myomectomy (a fibroid removal operation) to remove the individual fibroid(s) that might prevent pregnancy. While myomectomies don't resolve the problem forever—fibroids tend to come back, pesky little buggers that they are—removing fibroids can improve your fertility long enough to get you a baby.

The downside to a myomectomy is that it requires a large incision across your lower abdomen, so you'll have to stay in the hospital for a fairly lengthy recuperation. (One of my friends who had this procedure had to take more than a month off from work. For some of us this is a blessing; for others it isn't such a great thing.) Newer techniques such as uterine artery embolization (a catheter is inserted through an artery in your leg and used to cut off blood supply to the fibroid), cryomyolysis (the fibroid is frozen), and myolysis (an electric current is used to cut off blood supply to the fibroid) are promising new ways to treat fibroids with less invasive surgery. Discuss your options with your doctor; if necessary, search out a surgeon who can perform the right procedure for your needs.

You also can take drugs that shut down the hormone support for the fibroid. These drugs are often prescribed before surgery to stop the growth of the fibroid and hopefully shrink it at least a little. The drugs most commonly used are Lupron and Synarel (you can read more about these meds in chapter 11, although the dosage differs from that given to IVF patients). Lupron prevents you from making estradiol, which is what the fibroid thrives upon. Without the estradiol, the fibroid should shrink and your symptoms should diminish. These drugs also shut down your menstrual cycle, so you won't get a period. If you have anemia from all the bleeding your fibroid has caused, not getting your period for a while will enable you to recover. This may be important before major surgery. However, once you go off the meds, the fibroid will start growing, often faster than before.

# Luteal Phase Defect (LPD)

**What it is:** The luteal phase is the second half of your menstrual cycle, the time between ovulation and the start of your period. This is the critical time when your corpus luteum produces the progesterone your body needs to develop and ripen the uterine lining (the endometrium) and to support a beginning pregnancy. The corpus luteum is what is left after the follicle ruptures when it releases an egg during ovulation. If your corpus luteum isn't able to provide sufficient progesterone, your uterine lining may not be sufficiently developed to support embryo implantation. The lining must develop at precisely the right rate to be ready to support an embryo. Some doctors believe that a lining even a day behind in development can preclude a pregnancy from progressing. Alternatively, your lining may be sufficiently developed but your corpus luteum is not making enough progesterone to meet the needs of the developing fetus, and you're at higher risk of miscarriage. The failure of the corpus luteum to make sufficient progesterone is known as a luteal phase defect or LPD.

It is easily diagnosed and fixed. A blood test taken just before your period (about three days before) can tell your doctor whether you're making enough progesterone. For a more thorough diagnosis, your doctor may do an endometrial biopsy. The results can tell her how in sync the development of your lining is compared to the time in the cycle when the biopsy is taken.

**Treatment:** If you're not making enough progesterone, your RE may prescribe progesterone support (suppositories are most common) to take either after you ovulate or after a pregnancy has been detected. Alternatively, she may give you a medication like Clomid to help strengthen your ovulation and improve the function of your corpus luteum.

If you're already undergoing more advanced fertility treatment like

IUI or IVF, progesterone support will automatically be prescribed, so you probably don't need to worry about LPD. The nice thing about most assisted reproductive technologies is that they leave nothing to chance, and virtually every possible "weakness" in your system will be corrected, including the possibility that there isn't enough progesterone to develop your uterine lining and to support an early pregnancy.

LPD is one of those things that is an easy fix and hopefully, once diagnosed and treated, will allow you to achieve a healthy full-term pregnancy.

# Polycystic Ovarian Syndrome (PCO, PCOS, Stein-Leventhal Syndrome, Syndrome X, and Syndrome O)

**What it is:** Polycystic ovarian syndrome (hereinafter PCOS no matter how many names it may have) is an extremely complex and poorly understood syndrome that affects ovulation. Basically, your endocrine system is out of whack and you don't ovulate effectively. Because of certain hormone imbalances, you produce a lot of immature eggs every month. REs love comparing ovaries and the reproductive system to cars (this analogy is discussed in greater detail in the section on premature ovarian failure) but for now, think of women with PCOS as having ovaries like little Porsches. PCOS isn't just a risk factor for infertility, but in more severe cases it poses long-term health problems, predisposing you to type II diabetes and heart disease.

There are many symptoms of PCOS, and the presence of one may make your doctor suspect the syndrome, but she cannot diagnose it conclusively unless you have at least a couple of symptoms. Symptoms that may point to PCOS include irregular periods or complete lack of periods; weight gain or carrying extra weight around your midsection (including obesity); acne; excessive facial hair; infertility; high blood pressure; elevated cholesterol levels; dark patches of skin on the back of the neck, arms, breasts, and between the thighs; skin tags; insulin resistance (a condition similar to and perhaps a precursor of diabetes), and chronic pelvic pain. (What a lovely list of symptoms. *Not!*) Never thought the symptoms were related? Join the club; some doctors don't even figure it out (nice, eh?).

Syndrome X is very similar to PCOS and shows many of the same characteristics. The primary difference between PCOS and syndrome X is that to be diagnosed with syndrome X, you *must* have certain conditions (insulin resistance or diabetes, and high blood pressure, and obesity, and high cholesterol) at the same time. Another significant difference between syndrome X and PCOS is that men can have syndrome X. I will hereafter refer to PCOS and syndrome X interchangeably, even though they are not—strictly speaking—the same thing.

The cause of PCOS is unknown, but recent research suggests a genetic component and some kind of relationship with the body's ability to metabolize insulin. High levels of insulin (insulin resistance) can inhibit the ovulatory system and affect fat and sugar metabolism (thus explaining why so many women with PCOS are overweight and at high risk for developing type II diabetes). PCOS usually is diagnosed after testing various hormone levels, cholesterol levels, thyroid function, blood sugar levels, and having an ultrasound examination of your ovaries.

If you suspect you've got PCOS and want to get pregnant, you need to see a reproductive endocrinologist (RE) as these folks have received the most training in delicately balancing the many hormones (including male hormones) that are out of whack when you have PCOS. Your workup should include blood tests to determine:

- Your LH:FSH ratio (when the LH is higher than the FSH, you may have PCOS).

- Your testosterone level. (Okay, hold on, lots of big words coming your way! Don't worry too much if you can't pronounce them, neither can most people!)

- Your DHEAS level (dehydroepiandrosterone sulfate).

- Your androstenedione level.

- Your SHBG level (sex hormone binding globulin).

- Your prolactin level.

- Your TSH level (thyroid stimulating hormone).

- A fasting comprehensive lipid panel (cholesterol, triglycerides, and c-peptide).

- An IGTT level (fasting insulin).

- An ultrasound of your ovaries (looking for signs of Porsche-like activity, lots of small follicles).

**Treatment:** Treating PCOS should become your priority in terms of family building and for your long-term health, especially when your PCOS is *severe*. Current research suggests that PCOS puts you at risk of developing type II diabetes, high blood pressure, heart disease, thyroid disease, and endometrial cancer. So, even if you're not trying to get pregnant, you should monitor your thyroid function, blood sugar, insulin, and cholesterol levels regularly (once a year).

Once you've determined how severe your PCOS is, you can discuss with your RE whether to proceed with lifestyle changes and old-fashioned pregnancy efforts (sex) or more aggressive drug treatments to treat the PCOS and, hopefully, get you pregnant. If you're insulin resistant, using medication like metformin (Glucophage) may restore normal ovulatory function. Dietary changes (going on a low-carbohydrate diet under the supervision of a nutritionist) and exercise are also very beneficial. I know one woman who was diagnosed with marked insulin resistance. She began a rigorous exercise schedule and consulted a nutritionist instead of taking medication. About a year later, she started trying to conceive the old-fashioned way and conceived the first month she tried.

Many doctors recommend trying medication and lifestyle changes together for the greatest and fastest results.

PCOS may also mean that the quality of your eggs is impaired (this is not true for all women with PCOS). Doctors are constantly looking for ways to improve egg quality in women with PCOS. Metformin and other insulin sensitizing drugs that regulate certain hormones may be helpful. (It's believed that insulin resistance throws your hormonal system out of whack.) As of this writing, there's no research data that prove that insulin-sensitizing medications improve egg quality in women undergoing IVF. Anecdotal evidence, however, suggests that taking these drugs can increase the number of mature eggs retrieved during an IVF cycle. Additionally, as women with PCOS tend to have lower progesterone levels after ovulation, they'll probably get progesterone support during the luteal phase of their cycle. This is normal practice during IUI and IVF cycles, but doctors often prescribe progesterone support for women with PCOS trying to conceive without ART.

Other treatments for PCOS include ovarian surgery, either ovarian drilling (exactly like what it sounds, they drill a hole in your ovary), or something called a wedge resection (where they take a wedgelike slice out of your ovary and stitch it back up; this is thought to reduce the number of potential follicles in your ovary and reduce hormone levels). Neither of these treatments is terribly effective (some studies report success below 25 percent for ovarian drilling), and with the advent of co-culture programs and assisted hatching (see chapters 7 and 12) that improve egg and embryo quality during IVF, it may be wiser to forgo expensive and painful surgery in favor of IVF. These treatments aren't cutting edge anymore; if you've got a doctor recommending that you try one of these procedures, consider getting a second opinion.

One last thing you should know about PCOS is that studies indicate that women with the syndrome have a 45 percent risk of miscarriage. Researchers have yet to figure out why this is true. Metformin use during treatment and the first trimester of pregnancy together with baby aspirin (an increasingly popular treatment for pregnancy loss) has shown a marked reduction in miscarriage among the PCOS population.

# Premature Ovarian Failure, High FSH, and Poor Responders

**What it is:** I lump these three diagnoses together because in each your ovaries aren't gonna do what you want them to, and that's make eggs to make babies.

The one thing we all know—or should know—about our bodies and our ovaries is that they are time bombs; the proverbial biological clock isn't a joke. As fetuses we all start with millions of eggs in our ovaries. But by the time we're babies, the number is down to the hundreds of thousands, and it diminishes every year. We lose something like 1,000 potential eggs every month from natural attrition (and if you smoke, the nicotine kills the eggs off even faster). As we veer toward thirty-five— and hit the fertility land mine—we're dealing with seriously reduced quantities of usable eggs. Men have millions of sperm until the day they die, and we get this constant reduction in our fertility. *It ain't fair!* But for some women life is even harsher.

Some women hit menopause at thirty; that's what premature ovarian failure (POF) is. Anyone under the age of forty (another fertility benchmark) with a vastly diminished supply of eggs is experiencing POF. Women with POF are also at risk for certain autoimmune disorders (thyroid and adrenal issues are most common), so getting diagnosed can be important for long-term health management. Since you can't look inside and count your eggs every month, you might be wondering how you tell if you're in POF or heading that way. One sure sign something is wrong is that your period is irregular or nonexistent. Another indication of your diminishing fertility is discovered through blood tests.

Remember that CD3 blood work your RE performs as part of your initial workup? She is checking the level of two hormones, follicle stimulating hormone (FSH) and estradiol (E2). I go into greater detail about these two hormones in chapter 11 and in the Appendix, but for women with POF, these hormones play a great big role in your infertility. If you're not interested in how it all works, skip ahead and ignore the next couple of paragraphs.

Your body makes FSH to tell your ovaries to start making eggs. As your body starts making eggs, your ovaries tell your brain to make estradiol. The eggs will now grow from the estradiol, not from the FSH. The presence of estradiol in your body tells your brain that it can shut down the production of FSH. The levels of these two hormones are interdependent; FSH leads to estradiol production and the estradiol in turn shuts down the production of FSH. This is called a feedback loop, and it's discussed in great detail in the Appendix.

Many doctors liken FSH to the gas in a car (back to the car analogies), telling the car to go faster. As you step on the gas, your FSH level should rise, and you should make eggs. As you make the eggs, your estradiol level rises and that becomes the brake telling the car to slow down. The problem is that in women with premature ovarian failure, your body doesn't respond the way it should to high levels of FSH by making eggs, and it doesn't get the signal from rising estradiol levels to shut down the production of FSH. FSH levels stay elevated all the time; the pedal is to the metal all the time (to continue the car analogy).

When your RE sees an elevated FSH level, she knows that the feedback loop isn't working properly, which generally means that something is going haywire with your egg production. Usually, it means you're in POF, and your eggs aren't developing normally.

This blood work may also show (instead of or in addition to high FSH levels) elevated levels of E2 at the beginning of the cycle. The estradiol level may stay elevated throughout the cycle in a continuing effort to shut down production of FSH and artificially suppress the level of FSH your body is making; continuous high E2 levels may mask high FSH.

Now I'm not going to tell you what normal levels are. FSH and E2 levels are lab specific. Every lab has attributed certain values to the numbers it gets from the FSH and E2 tests it runs, and no two labs ever come up with the same value. Some find anything under 8 to be a normal FSH level, while others say anything under 14 is normal. Only your doctor can tell you the range of specific values she is looking for from the lab she uses. Your prior results are meaningless unless they are from the same lab.

FSH results fluctuate among all women, so if you do get a high result once, your RE likely will have you come back for repeat blood work. The bad news is that it's not a good thing to have consistently high levels. The good news is that the second time you come back the results might be lower, and that may mean your ovaries aren't in complete retirement (at least they haven't moved to Florida yet). You might respond better to IVF stimulation during a cycle in which your hormone levels are a little lower than in the past; fluctuating levels can sometimes provide windows of opportunity for better egg recruitment. But many doctors believe that one high FSH test is ominous and is predictive of potential poor response to treatment, no matter what later blood tests may reveal.

To confirm your blood test results from the beginning of your menstrual cycle your RE may have you take the Clomid challenge test. Don't worry, you don't need a sports bra for this. Your blood will be drawn on the third day of your menstrual cycle (CD3); on CD5 you'll begin taking Clomid, a medication that causes you to ovulate. You will take the medication for five days and go back for more blood work on CD10. A normal test result would look something like this:

CD3: low FSH and E2 (estradiol)
CD10: low FSH, higher/rising E2

Your FSH should be low on CD10 because your body has already started producing eggs, your E2 level has risen, and that has told your body to shut off FSH production by this point in time (that feedback loop is working). An abnormal result might look something like this:

CD3: high FSH and E2
CD10: high FSH, higher/rising E2

Or

CD3: low FSH and high E2

CD10: high FSH, higher/rising E2

The advantage of the Clomid challenge test is that it more accurately identifies diminished ovarian reserve than the CD3 blood work. Poor FSH levels on CD10 are as important as those on CD3. FSH levels on CD10 help your doctor determine whether your FSH was artificially low on CD3 due to abnormally high E2 levels at the beginning of the cycle or was the bottom part of a normal fluctuating cycle. The Clomid challenge test helps your doctor conclusively determine whether you have FSH issues or problems with your ovaries' ability to produce eggs in response to hormonal stimulation. This helps her decide which type of treatment will best work to get you pregnant.

Lastly, for reasons doctors still don't understand, some women pass all these tests but don't respond to treatment and don't produce sufficient quantities of healthy eggs to achieve pregnancy. This is the poor responder without high FSH that I mentioned earlier. In a young woman this is perplexing, in a woman over thirty-five it's assumed the poor response is due to "advanced maternal age." (I really hate this diagnosis. Would any sane person outside of Hollywood ever describe a thirty-five-year-old as having "advanced age"?)

**Treatment:** Whatever the cause of your ovarian failure, my heart goes out to you. Doctors haven't figured out how to turn back the biological clock. But they're working on it. And that's not to say you won't get pregnant; women with ovarian reserve/response issues do get pregnant. But success rates for women with POF undergoing standard IVF are pretty depressing; fewer than 5 percent get pregnant. Because success rates are so low, many clinics won't even attempt to treat high FSH patients.

Some clinics work with high FSH patients with some success. If you decide to go this route, look for a clinic with a state-of-the art coculture program (a special culture medium that is used to help nourish embryos as they grow, some clinics even use your endometrial tissue in the culture medium) as this may help improve embryo quality (I talk more about coculture programs in chapter 7). You also may try on your own as your chances of conceiving—depending on how highly elevated your FSH is—are about the same with and without treatment.

If you receive this diagnosis and don't like the success rate for conventional IVF, you've still got one very good option: use donor eggs. No matter your age (the one good thing is that the uterus doesn't age) with this diagnosis, ovum donation is an extremely successful option (see chapter 7). And I mean, *extremely* successful. Your chances of conceiving with donor eggs are probably better than they would be if you used your own eggs from when you were twenty-seven. With ovum donation your success rate may be closer to 50 percent than 5 percent.

Additionally, many women have found changing their diet and using acupuncture helps them get pregnant with high FSH. Wheat grass juice (which has been shown to lower FSH levels) might be a good place for patients with high FSH to start. Most physicians don't believe that these nutritional changes make a real difference. Tell that to a woman with high FSH who got pregnant after she changed her diet! It's hard to know what really helps.

Cytoplasm transfer offers another treatment option for women with egg quality issues. This newly emerging technique (which is still experimental) takes DNA from your egg and places it inside the nutrient components of a donor's egg (essentially your DNA goes in a healthy egg). It is a promising new frontier in reproductive science and offers potential hope to many women with ovarian reserve/response issues. Lastly, some doctors are trying natural cycle IVF for women with ovarian reserve problems (discussed in greater detail in chapter 7) and having modest success.

Unfortunately, today the options and outcome for women with these diagnoses is still extremely limited. Don't give up hope, do your research, be your own advocate, and *go for it!* Women with these issues can and do get pregnant, you could be one of them!

## Recurrent Pregnancy Loss and IVF Failure

**What it is:** For me, this may be the most important section of this book. My biggest problem seems to have something to do with my body's overzealous ability to form blood clots at the site of implantation and with my autoimmune system's response to pregnancy. One of the newest areas of research in reproductive medicine is focusing on how bodies—immune systems—respond to pregnancy. If you're not getting pregnant after multiple IVF cycles (with good egg and embryo quality) or are experiencing multiple miscarriages your body may be responding to pregnancy in an abnormal way. Check out chapter 4 if you want even more detail about what's involved in this immune response.

**Treatment:** There is a lot more information about treatment for IVF failure and recurrent pregnancy loss than there used to be, but it's still very hard to find the information you need. And, when you do find it, it's often in medical jargon that's incomprehensible to those who don't have advanced medical degrees. There's a lot of controversy about this stuff, and not a lot of studies that prove that treating reproductive immune disorders is helpful. But talk to patients who've been treated for a reproductive immune disorder, and you'll hear a different story.

This can be incredibly boring stuff to read. I'm going break it down for you as I did in chapter 4 and will try to oversimplify everything. If you need more specific information about these treatments, check out the Resources section (see Reproductive Immunologists).

### BLOOD-CLOTTING DISORDERS

If you're diagnosed with either an inherited or acquired blood-clotting disorder—like an MTHFR mutation or APA (antiphospholipid antibodies)—most doctors recommend treatment with heparin, an injectable blood thinner (also known as an anticoagulant). Some physicians feel strongly that low molecular weight heparin (Lovenox) is more effective than standard heparin therapy. Others feel that heparin therapy is more effective. (See what I mean about controversial?) You'll probably also be told to take one baby aspirin (81 mg) every day. Treatment begins either at the beginning of your menstrual cycle or shortly after ovulation/egg retrieval and, if you get pregnant, usually continues until six weeks after your baby is born. Heparin is not dangerous to a developing fetus and is not excreted in breast milk. But extended heparin therapy can cause a reduction in bone mass and put you at higher risk for osteoporosis. Before you take heparin, discuss these risks with your doctor and find out whether you might consider supplemental calcium and/or having a baseline bone density study.

More intensive therapies are available for women who fail to respond to heparin therapy. One alternative treatment involves prednisone. Many physicians, however, don't like to use it because it causes an increased risk of complications during pregnancy. There also is an intravenous treatment available, known as IVIG or IVGG (the tongue-twisting version is intravenous immunoglobulin or gammaglobulin). IVIG is *expensive* and unpleasant to administer (it can make you feel like you have the worst flu of your life). I will talk more about IVIG in a moment.

Current statistics indicate that the live birth rate for most of these conditions, when treated, is around 70 percent. Multiple miscarriages before treatment reduce your chances of success, especially if you've had more than five losses. If you're pregnant and have a history of recurrent pregnancy loss, it's not too late to get tested. Repeat and initial testing during pregnancy is recommended for patients with prior loss and/or a positive antibody test.

Scientists have only recently discovered that thrombophilias play a role in reproductive failure. There is limited research suggesting that treatments such as heparin therapy are effective (and that the live birth rate is really 70 percent). A recent study in the journal *Fertility and Sterility* concluded that women with some of these conditions (homozygosity for MTHFR included) are just as likely to carry to term whether they are treated with heparin, Lovenox, baby aspirin, or nothing at all.

## THE BABY-KILLING CELLS

If you have an issue with HLA compatibility (where your HLA and your partner's HLA are similar), treatment will attempt to immunize the mother with the father's white blood cells in the hope that her body recognizes the different HLA and starts making blocking antibodies. The treatment is called LIT, short for lymphocyte (a type of white blood cell) immune therapy. The injections start before pregnancy is attempted, and, if all goes well, continue during the pregnancy. LIT therapy isn't widely available, and the FDA recently temporarily stopped LIT administration and notified physicians treating patients with LIT that they would have to comply with special approval procedures for new drug applications before treatment could resume.

To ensure that no blood-borne illnesses are transmitted from the injection, it's important that your partner's blood be tested for certain diseases before LIT therapy is administered. Assuming he's healthy, the risks associated with this treatment are pretty low; the most frequent side effect is a rash at the injection site. Another option in treating a problem with these blocking antibodies is to undergo intravenous treatment with IVIG. If you've been diagnosed with elevated NK cells or cytokines (the embryotoxic cells), IVIG is the therapy of choice.

IVIG is a blood product taken from people without any immune disorders that contains normal levels of blocking and other antibodies that should help protect the fetus. IVIG is very expensive (up to $2,500 per intravenous infusion) and is used to treat reproductive disorders on an experimental basis. Absent a diagnosis for a nonreproductive disorder, it's not covered by most insurance. Reproductive treatment with IVIG is under review by the FDA and hopefully will be covered in the future. IVIG is administered intravenously, and a nurse must administer the infusion, usually in a hospital. You can arrange to do it at home after the initial infusion in a hospital. Side effects are much more severe than those caused by LIT and are more common (they include migrainelike headaches and severe flulike symptoms). A single treatment with IVIG generally is not sufficient. Expect to undergo intravenous treatment sometimes every month of a full-term pregnancy. At $2,500 a pop, this can get overwhelmingly expensive.

There isn't a lot of good, solid research to prove how effective these therapies are. Reproductive immunology (I've got to say it again) is cutting-edge science. Carolyn Coulam, M.D., is a leading reproductive immunologist and has extensively studied IVIG therapy. Her research—perhaps the only really reliable research to date—suggests that preconception treatment with IVIG can increase the live birth rate to 80 percent. LIT therapy has shown a live birth rate of about 60 percent, a 10 percent improvement over the live birth rate without treatment, which is 50 percent.

You might be wondering why there isn't more reliable research on this stuff. Let me ask you this: would you participate in a research study if there was a chance you'd be in the control group (receiving no treatment) or the group receiving placebo treatment and might miscarry again? I wouldn't take that kind of chance. It's hard to risk losing another baby in the name of science. But it's easy to try an experimental therapy, even if it might not work for you. This is what my friend Laura and I did.

We met while undergoing IVF. We soon realized that we both experienced recurrent pregnancy losses and had the same immune diagnosis (MTHFR). We forged a fast bond, went through cycles together, and even experienced miscarriages within days of each other. At the recommendation of our respective reproductive immunologists, Laura and I decided to undergo different treatments for recurrent pregnancy loss.

In addition to the prescription blood thinners that we were already taking, Laura decided to try lymphocyte immune therapy (LIT), and I did IVIG. Laura tolerated the LIT well. I didn't get off so well. The first administration of IVIG was brutal. I was violently ill with severe flulike symptoms the night and day after the infusion. I had the first infusion in a hospital setting and arranged for a home health care nurse to do the other infusions at home. I didn't have as many side effects after the second and third infusions, but still felt pretty lousy afterward.

After numerous losses, Laura successfully carried triplets to term with

LIT (you go, girl!). I got pregnant at the same time as Laura and then miscarried. Neither of us will ever know for sure if these treatments really helped us. But we both feel that the prescription blood thinners were important in helping us maintain a pregnancy. Laura feels strongly that her LIT played a role in her achieving a full term pregnancy. I haven't been able to carry to term, but I still believe this is an important area of reproductive science.

## Unexplained Infertility

**What it is:** If you've been through all the tests and done a couple of IVF cycles and your RE still can't explain why you're not conceiving (and this means she excludes vague diagnoses like "advanced maternal age"), life pretty much just stinks. I am so sorry. This is a very frustrating place to be; not having answers is the *worst!*

However, one thing to keep in mind about infertility treatment is that "unexplained infertility" cannot be diagnosed without IVF. IVF serves diagnostic purposes for many couples because it reveals problems that aren't otherwise detected (see chapter 7). If you haven't gotten pregnant after repeated IVF attempts and there appears to be no problem with your egg, sperm, embryo, and uterus, then you fall into the true definition of unexplained infertility. If you're told that there's nothing wrong with you (and you have unexplained infertility) but you haven't tried IVF, check out chapter 7 and read about why you should try IVF.

Perhaps children really do pick their time to come into this world, and it doesn't matter how long or hard we try to conceive; they come when they're ready and not a moment before. Perhaps stress plays a greater role than science understands. All those people who've gone through treatment for years, then decide to adopt and are later surprised with a pregnancy suggest that stress and happiness play big roles in the conception process. But then how do we explain the completely stressed-out and depressed workaholic who accidentally gets pregnant?

**Treatment:** If no one can explain your infertility (even after IVF and an immune workup) and you want to keep trying, I recommend looking at alternative therapies. I have heard of countless women—and even know some—who went to homeopaths and acupuncturists, hypnotists, stress-management therapists, and other healers and became pregnant after more conventional therapies failed them.

But my heart goes out to you. I don't know why I can't carry a baby to term. I've made my peace with my body, but without a real explanation, the subject remains open. Should I look into treatment again? Will science discover something that will help me? Even now when I've got this beautiful baby boy, I'm frustrated and confused. It's terrible not knowing why you can't have a baby; *it just plain sucks!*

# 6

## Calling All Men

Actually, infertility affects a lot of men. Statistics suggest that men are implicated in up to 40 to 50 percent of all cases of infertility. That's a pretty huge statistic; it's something like 2.5 million men every year. Male-factor infertility can be boring and complicated, sometimes mind-numbingly so. The white lab coat is on again, so bear with me if I lose my sense of humor occasionally in this chapter. Healthy sperm play an important role in getting you pregnant, and I don't want to short-shrift you in the info department. Some of this stuff is also a little graphic (it's those needles again!); I'll warn you before we get to a discussion that might freak you and/or your partner out. You might want to wait to read these sections until you know that you're dealing with the relevant medical issue rather than experience unnecessary needle-related anxiety.

Most of the time the remedy for male factor is simple (women aren't so lucky). Lifestyle and dietary changes, ICSI (in which the sperm is injected into the egg to achieve fertilization), or other procedures usually work to treat men's fertility problems. There also are surgical procedures that can help a man with *no sperm* in his ejaculate father a biological child (wow!). Would that REs could help women find a healthy egg in their ovaries the way a urologist can find sperm in men's testes. I sometimes think that Mother Nature is both ageist and sexist when it comes to fertility. (Who decided she was a *woman* anyway? Seems like a man was responsible for these things to me!)

Though in many cases male factor is often easily treatable, it can cause considerable problems, especially because many men become withdrawn and uncommunicative when their manhood is called into question. We'll talk about how to help your husband or partner through this crisis in a few pages, but let's start with the basics first. How much sperm do you really need to get pregnant?

All you really need is one good, healthy sperm to get the job done. The question is whether the sperm is available through a normal ejaculatory process and good, old-fashioned sex, whether you'll need to use ICSI (where the sperm is injected into the egg to achieve fertilization), or whether you need microsurgery to find the sperm in your partner's testes and then use ICSI. But please do keep this in mind: *all you need is one*.

First things first: you need to find out if you've got a good one in there somewhere!

## Urologists and Semen Analyses

Men should be tested before or at the same time that you're getting tested. Your husband is just as likely as you are to be the cause (or part of the cause) of your inability to conceive, so there is no point in waiting to have him checked out. Even though he's going to complain about getting tested, you may spend a lot less time in treatment if he's got an easily treatable problem. Some couples find out they don't need sophisticated reproductive help once they've dealt with the male-factor issue. Your first stop should be a urologist's office, and preferably one that specializes in infertility. Check out ASRM, RESOLVE, or AIA for a reference if you can't get one from your doctor.

Your second step should be to schedule at least two semen analyses over a period of weeks (let your urologist tell you his preference for timing). Oftentimes, you need to compare the results of one semen sample with another to determine if there's really a problem (flukes do happen). Each semen sample should be obtained after two to five days of abstinence and analyzed within two hours of collection. Your third step is for your husband or partner to have a good physical examination with the urologist.

The physical exam should include a complete medical and sexual history, an examination of his testicles after they have been warmed (usually on a heating pad, as this makes physical abnormalities easier to identify), an examination of the rest of his body and reproductive organs (including a rectal exam to examine his prostate), and blood work to evaluate his hormone levels (testosterone, FSH, LH, and prolactin). Ultrasound studies may be ordered to help visualize the interior reproductive structures, including a transrectal ultrasound procedure. (Hey, his workup has something as potentially uncomfortable and embarrassing as the many unpleasant diagnostic tests we get to go through! Mother Nature may be a woman after all!) His urologist may also want to examine the inside of these organs (think of this as the male version of the HSG) using contrast dye and an X-ray machine.

The medical history helps identify risk factors for male infertility. Risk factors include a history of prostatitis or genital infection, testicular trauma, early onset or delayed onset of puberty, exposure to toxic substances (lead, X rays, mercury, and other chemicals and radioactive substances), cigarette or marijuana use, heavy alcohol consumption, mumps after puberty, DES exposure by his mother, certain prescription medications (for ulcers and psoriasis), hernia repair, exposure of the testes to high temperatures (hot tubs, tighty whities, frequent bicycle riding), and cystic fibrosis (even carrying the gene for cystic fibrosis). The sexual history helps identify sexually transmitted diseases that could implicate fertility issues, as well as ejaculatory problems and hormonal imbalances. The physical exam can diagnose a varicoceles (an enlargement of the testicular veins that may cause infertility from increased heat in the testes); blockages that impair the flow of seminal fluid; small, soft testicles that suggest problems with sperm production; problems with the epididymis (the place where sperm is stored); and an enlarged prostate, which can contribute fluid to the semen volume.

Blood tests check for hormone imbalances that can affect the development of the sperm. An elevated FSH level and/or decreased testicular volume can indicate problems with sperm production. For example, the lack of FSH and LH may indicate that your partner has Kallman's syndrome, a congenital disorder in which the hypothalamus fails to tell the body to make the hormones necessary to make sperm. Although fewer than 5 percent of men have a hormone imbalance that can be treated with hormone therapy, your urologist may recommend drug therapy to help balance these hormones.

Certain gene mutations also can be detected through blood tests and can reveal the cause of poor sperm counts. Klinefelter's syndrome occurs in men with an extra X chromosome, which renders him sterile (instead of the normal 46XY chromosomal complement, a man with Klinefelter's has 47XXY). Men with cystic fibrosis or who carry the mutation for cystic fibrosis often have a congenital malformation of the vas deferens (known as CAV) that causes something known as azoospermia (no sperm in the seminal fluid). This can be treated with surgical sperm retrieval and IVF with ICSI. Recently, researchers discovered that a mutation on the Y chromosome inhibits or stops sperm production. While it's possible to achieve a pregnancy with this condition, it's hereditary, so you pass the potential for infertility along to your son. Knowing you have this mutation enables you to make informed decisions about whether or not you want to pass this and other defects on to your child.

Ninety percent of the time, a thorough exam will point to a diagnosis. Additional testing will help your urologist confirm the diagnosis and determine a treatment plan. Relying solely on the results of a semen analysis often fails to identify a treatable cause of infertility. Having an exam and undergoing some additional testing may help you avoid using sophisticated assisted reproductive technologies. For example, a urologist can treat your partner for something like a varicoceles (which might explain a low semen count) and help you achieve conception the old-fashioned way. But what about the semen analysis? What does it really tell you?

Most semen analyses are performed and analyzed in accordance with World Health Organization (WHO) standards. A stricter standard, called a Kruger analysis, may be used to assess sperm shape. Under WHO standards, the lab examines your husband's semen sample for semen volume count (the amount of sperm contained in a certain volume of fluid, also known as sperm density or sperm concentration), size and shape (morphology), and ability to move (motility).

According to World Health Organization 1992 standards, normal seminal fluid volume (the amount of fluid present in the sample) ranges between two and six milliliters with a concentration of greater than twenty million sperm per milliliter (in other words, there should be twenty million sperm for every volume of fluid produced). A normal sperm count per WHO standards has greater than forty million sperm per sample (roughly twenty million sperm in two milliliters of fluid). More than 50 percent of the sperm must be alive and moving for the sample to have normal motility. Normal morphology requires that more than 30 percent of the sperm have a normal shape. The viscosity of the fluid (ejaculate normally liquefies within an hour and does not show sperm clumping) will be examined as will the white blood cell count. Some white blood cells are normal in seminal fluid, but an excessive quantity could indicate an infection. Finally, the pH of the seminal fluid should be between seven and eight.

If morphology is assessed by strict Kruger criteria, more than 12 percent of the sperm must be shaped normally for a man to be considered fertile. The Kruger analysis examines 200 or more sperm on a stained slide at $1,000 \times$ magnification. The length, width, and shape of the sperm head, nucleus, midpiece, and tail are all examined for defects or irregularities. Less than 5 percent normal morphology predicts an extremely low fertilization potential without assistance from ICSI. And by the way, it is possible to get a normal morphology report from a semen analysis performed in accordance with WHO reference standards and get a frighteningly low Kruger report. Because morphology is so important to fertilization, there are some other tests you may want to have performed when you're facing male infertility due to poor morphology. I'll get to these other sperm tests in a second, but first I want to talk about the problems with interpreting semen analyses.

Recently, the general criteria for judging semen have been called into question by the National Institute of Child Health and Human Development Reproductive Medicine Network. NIH has proposed that a sperm count greater than forty-eight million sperm per milliliter (a difference of twenty-eight million from the WHO standards), more than 63 percent motile sperm (a 13 percent difference), and a strict Kruger morphology of 12 percent or greater (a completely different standard, as WHO doesn't use the Kruger standard) is more likely than WHO standards to predict fertilization potential.

Another factor that throws a wrench into interpreting results is that the lab that analyzes your sample may use different parameters altogether. Your lab may use regional guidelines for where you live or may use different numbers. For example, many labs in the New York metropolitan area consider sixty million sperm per milliliter to be ideal. But Midwestern labs may assess sperm using a reference value of twenty million sperm per milliliter. Are men in New York more virile than men elsewhere in the country? Or is one of these standards just whacked? More confusing still, when looking at motility, some labs look only at the overall forward progression of the sperm across the microscope slide, while other labs score a collection of individual sperm on their motility and then total the numbers to assess an average motility score. Under the latter system, the higher the score is above an established reference number, the more normal the motility of the sperm.

Morphology can get even crazier. The Kruger reference looks for 12 percent normally shaped sperm, WHO looks for 30 percent or more normally shaped sperm, and some labs look for more than 80 percent normal forms. And, of course, it is possible to get a normal result using WHO standards and a grossly abnormal result based on the Kruger criteria.

There is also a gray area in which semen analyses are neither normal nor abnormal. With the standards proposed by NIH, the gray area encompasses a sperm count between 13.5 and 48 million sperm (that's kind of a big range, don't you think?), motility between 32 percent and 63 percent, and morphology between 9 percent and 12 percent (using Kruger standards). Do you treat a man with a semen analysis in this range or not? Who's to say what's right and what's wrong, what's infertile and what's fertile?

And none of this explains how Charlie, with his seriously defective 0 percent normally shaped sperm, managed to get me pregnant without any infertility treatment. Doctors admit it's not uncommon for a man who is told he's infertile to get you pregnant without any medical assistance. As I said before, all you need is one healthy sperm.

If your partner does get results that place him in a gray area where it's unclear whether you'd benefit from techniques like ICSI, there are additional tests that can help you make a treatment plan. If, for example, you've gotten morphology results that are unclear, a sperm penetration assay (SPA) can be performed to assess the sperm's ability to penetrate a hamster's egg. In about 80 percent of cases, SPA results accurately reflect the sperm's ability to penetrate your egg. This can help you determine whether morphology or other sperm issues are preventing you from achieving fertilization.

A good urologist who specializes in treating infertility will know how best to interpret your husband's results and how and when to treat him. Some doctors may see a low semen analysis and then find a varicocele during the physical exam. Clumping and other semen issues can be treated with vitamins (Proxeed) or prescription medication. A complete absence of sperm may be remedied with surgery and IVF. ICSI can help you achieve fertilization even with the most severe morphology issues. And donor insemination is always a viable option.

There are several diagnoses and tests—including sperm viability assays, postcoital tests, hypogonadotropic hypogonadism—that I don't include, as a full discussion of male-factor infertility is beyond the scope of this book. But I've listed sources for more information in the back of the book, and I encourage you to educate yourself using the Resources section, the World Wide Web, and your urologist. Certain male reproductive disorders also implicate long-term health issues, so I strongly suggest that you get a thorough workup with a good urologist.

Now let's discuss what you may be facing.

## ICSI (Intracytoplasmic Sperm Injection)

ICSI is often mentioned in my discussions of treatment for particular disorders, so let's talk about it first. ICSI is perhaps the biggest, most important advance in reproductive science in the last decade. It facilitates fertilization in cases where there is moderate to severe male-factor infertility and in cases where normal sperm are otherwise unable to penetrate the zona pellucida (the exterior shell of a woman's egg). Using this technique, doctors can isolate a single sperm from a semen sample (whether obtained from masturbation, surgery, cryopreservation, or a donor) and, using a microscope, inject it into an egg that has been harvested from a woman's body. Hopefully, fertilization will then take place in the proverbial petri dish used during IVF. However, there's no guarantee that even with ICSI, the sperm will fertilize the egg.

Fertilization occurs about 70 to 80 percent of the time with ICSI, but sometimes you'll luck out and get 100 percent fertilization (meaning all of your eggs are fertilized using the ICSI technique). Fertilization success rates with ICSI vary a lot based on the lab used and on the health of the sperm and egg selected. ICSI enables couples, who otherwise would've had to use donor sperm or adopt, to achieve a pregnancy. It often helps couples facing even the most severe male-factor infertility achieve a pregnancy. How cool is that?

ICSI has resulted in thousands of pregnancies and produced thousands of normal children, but there are risks you should be aware of. First of all, for reasons that researchers have yet to discover, the risk of conceiving identical twins (two genetically identical babies from one single egg) is higher with ICSI. Second, some studies report higher incidences of birth defects in children born from ICSI. Other studies, however, refute these findings. Still others show a link between ICSI and higher-than-average miscarriage rates. Research has yet to prove any of these theoretical links. Studies designed to explore the link between ICSI, birth defects, and miscarriages have only just begun.

If you're concerned about these risks, you might want to undergo preimplantation genetic diagnosis (PGD is discussed in greater detail in chapter 7) after you've achieved fertilization. PGD enables your embryologist to examine the genetic structure of an embryo to see if there are any potential DNA issues that might result in miscarriage or birth defects. PGD is not without risks (see chapter 7), however, so you should talk to your RE about whether it's warranted in your situation.

ICSI can also be used as a rescue technique after conventional IVF fertilization techniques have failed. That is, when the embryologist puts sperm and egg together and discovers that fertilization cannot take place without assistance. The embryologist may then want to try to achieve fertilization using ICSI. Rescue ICSI is far less successful than ICSI initiated soon after egg retrieval. But if you're undergoing IVF, rescue ICSI is an option you should know about and discuss with your doctors.

Now let's discuss some medical conditions that might warrant ICSI or more sophisticated surgeries.

## Anatomical Issues That Cause Problems with Sperm Production

### VARICOCELES

**What it is:** A varicocele is an enlarged vein in the testes. It usually occurs in the left testicle and develops during puberty. It is highly correlated with infertility, but doctors aren't certain how it impairs fertility. It is believed that the enlarged vein increases the blood flow and thus the heat to both testicles. Heat impairs sperm development. Although poor semen analyses aren't always caused by a varicocele, 90 percent of the time semen analyses from men with a varicocele show impaired sperm motility. Sixty-five percent of the time they manifest decreased sperm counts. Sperm morphology may also be abnormal.

Varicoceles are diagnosed during a urologist's exam. Some are so large they're visible; others can be felt only when your husband bears down as if to have a bowel movement while the scrotum is physically manipulated. Large varicoceles generally decrease sperm quality, but varicoceles of all sizes are a cause for concern.

**Treatment:** Treatment involves tying off certain veins in the testes in order to lower testicular temperature. (This is a very simplistic description of the procedure.) This can be accomplished microsurgically or radiographically. Complications occur when the vein(s) aren't tied off completely, and fluid collects in the testicle (called hydrocele). Using a skilled microsurgeon or experienced urologist is the best way to reduce your risk of complication. If you've already had surgery to correct a varicocele, radiographic procedures (where a balloon, coil, or other material is used to occlude the vein) may be preferable.

Sixty-five percent of men undergoing surgical varicocele repair will show improvements in their semen analysis about three months after the procedure is performed (usually sperm count improves the most). About 50 percent of couples who try to conceive naturally after a varicocele has been repaired will succeed. Having a varicocele repaired also can improve your chance of conceiving with IUI and IVF and can help you avoid using other surgical techniques to retrieve sperm from the testes.

However, varicocele repair will not correct severe problems with morphology. If your husband shows pronounced morphology problems, you'll need to use ICSI. Only your urologist can tell you whether it's worth having surgery to correct a varicocele, especially if you will still need to use ICSI after the surgery has been performed.

## CONGENITAL ABSENCE OF THE VAS DEFERENS
**What it is:** If the vas deferens (the ejaculatory duct) didn't form as your husband or partner was maturing, it's pretty much the same as having a

vasectomy. He's got sperm, they just can't get out of his reproductive tract.

**Treatment:** All hope is not lost; sperm can be obtained surgically. (We'll get to this in a moment.)

### HYPOSPADIAS

**What it is:** This is a condition that occurs when the opening of the urethra is in the wrong place. In this case, a man cannot deposit his sperm high enough in the vaginal canal to facilitate conception.

**Treatment:** This can be corrected surgically or through IUI.

### RETROGRADE EJACULATION

**What it is:** This often occurs in men with diabetes, who've had prostate surgery, or have neurological problems. In this case the seminal fluid travels down the ejaculatory duct but instead of flowing out through the urethra and the penis during orgasm, it flows backward into the bladder. This generally happens as a result of a weakened nerve that controls the bladder's sphincter muscle. Your husband or partner may have retrograde ejaculation if his test results show unusually low seminal fluid but good sperm count or when he notices that there's a milky look to his urine after orgasm. If there's sperm in your husband's urine, he probably suffers from retrograde ejaculation.

**Treatment:** Men with retrograde ejaculation may have sperm isolated from their urine or a bladder catheterization procedure followed by IUI.

### OTHER ANATOMICAL PROBLEMS CAUSED BY BLOCKAGES IN THE REPRODUCTIVE TRACT DUE TO INFECTION OR FROM A VASECTOMY

In this case, your husband makes sperm, but the sperm don't make it to the outside world due to an obstruction somewhere in the ejaculate's path. Fortunately, this can be overcome through reproductive surgery or more commonly now through the miscrosurgical removal of sperm.

Let's say you've seen a urologist and you've been told he's probably got sperm in there somewhere, but it isn't in his ejaculate. What do you do next?

## Surgery and Azoospermia

**What it is:** Next to ICSI, one of the most major advances in treatment for male infertility involves new microsurgical techniques for obtaining sperm from the testes and the epididymis (that's a tongue twister). When all other repairable or treatable causes of lack of sperm in the seminal fluid (azoospermia) have been ruled out, it's still possible to retrieve sperm— even immature, baby sperm—from the testes or epididymis to help achieve fertilization. Surgical removal of sperm enables you to use the best quality sperm possible during a cycle using ART. You can retrieve a sufficient number of sperm for immediate use and freeze some for subsequent use while minimizing damage to the reproductive tract (which may occur with reconstructive surgery) and jeopardizing additional attempts at surgical removal of his sperm.

**What's involved:** Before undergoing any attempt at surgical removal of sperm, your partner should have a complete genetic analysis performed. Certain chromosomal abnormalities may be the cause of his infertility and may be inheritable. If your urologist hasn't already had it done, a genetic workup (a karyotype analysis) and consultation with a genetic counselor are recommended. Not only are some of the conditions detected through a genetic workup inherited, but some of the chromosomal abnormalities mean that you're not likely to have successful surgical removal of sperm. At the very least, you want to know what your chances are for recovering usable, healthy sperm *before* you have the surgery.

Okay, here's your warning! Do not continue to read this section (skip ahead) if you've got an issue with needles (imagine my horror at having to write about this stuff?) or are in any way squeamish. Men should definitely think about holding off reading this stuff until their urologist mentions that they might benefit from one of these surgeries.

Depending on the specific cause of your husband's infertility, there are several options for surgically retrieving sperm. Once the sperm has been removed, ICSI will be used during an IVF cycle to help achieve fertilization. For men with obstructive azoospermia (where an obstruction in the male reproductive tract—for example, a problem with the vas deferens—makes it difficult if not impossible to ejaculate healthy quantities of sperm) surgical retrieval is an option in place of reconstructive surgery. In this case testicular fine needle aspiration (TFNA) may be your best bet at recovering sperm.

With TFNA, your husband is given a local anesthetic (and hopefully an IV sedative) and a puncture is made through the skin of the testes using a small-gauge needle connected to a syringe. The syringe is used to draw seminal fluid out of the testicle. Common complications of TFNA include hematomas and hematoceles (basically, this is just bruising in varying degrees of severity).

Percutaneous epididymal sperm aspiration (PESA) is another technique to retrieve sperm. PESA can be performed under local or general anesthesia. With this procedure, the surgeon holds the epididymis in between his thumb and forefinger and a needle (21-gauge butterfly needle, in case you're interested) attached to a syringe is inserted and then withdrawn until fluid can be seen entering the needle (much like when blood is drawn from your arm and the technician verifies that she has hit a vein by seeing the blood flow into the tube of the butterfly needle). The procedure is repeated until enough sperm has been removed. Depending on the individual patient and the skill of the surgeon, up to 20 percent of the time *insufficient* quantities of sperm are removed with PESA. Additionally, it's not uncommon for the sample to be contaminated with blood cells. This usually leads to decreased fertilization results and makes PESA a less-favored technique for retrieving sperm.

Two other techniques for patients with obstructive azoospermia are the percutaneous biopsy of the testis (PercBiopsy) and microsurgical epididymal sperm aspiration (MESA). In a PercBiopsy, greater quantities of sperm may be retrieved than with other techniques. In this procedure, a larger gauge needle gun (don't ask, cuz your husband doesn't want to know; see the Resources section if you're really interested in getting more information) is used under local anesthesia to remove the sperm from the testis. (Having seen a picture of this gun, I sure hope the local anesthesia includes some good sedatives.)

MESA, in contrast to all the other procedures I've discussed so far, is performed only under general anesthesia (thank god for small favors!). An incision is made in the testes and then, using a microscope, individual tubules of the epididymis (which contain sperm) are isolated. A needle is then used to aspirate and retrieve sperm directly from the epididymis. This procedure often produces large numbers of sperm and minimizes contamination with blood cells (one of the problems with PESA). Generally, very small quantities of fluid can be obtained, but that fluid contains a greater concentration of sperm than with the other techniques. One informal study compared TFNA, PercBiopsy, and MESA and concluded that MESA retrieved the greatest number of sperm with the highest motility, thus providing the best samples for ART and cryopreservation. Not every urologist, however, has the capabilities to perform this sophisticated procedure.

Nonobstructive azoospermia is where there is no sperm in the ejaculate due to severely abnormal sperm production. If you have nonobstructive azoospermia there are three options for surgical removal of sperm. Microdissection testicular sperm extraction (TESA), PercBiopsy (discussed above), and multiple standard biopsy. Both PercBiopsy and multiple standard biopsy come with high risks. PercBiopsy generally fails to yield sufficient quantities of sperm, and multiple standard biopsy may require the removal of a large volume of testicular tissue. In contrast, TESA improves sperm retrieval rates by almost 20 percent, and less testicular tissue is at risk of being removed. Success rates (live birth rates) for TESA attempts that successfully retrieved sperm were 40 percent. If you include those attempts that failed to yield any sperm, the success rate drops to 23 percent. Multiple TESA procedures are not recommended, as they can cause permanent changes in testicular function. If you're considering TESA, make sure you've got the best urological microsurgeon possible—someone with a lot of experience performing this procedure—to ensure the best results during a single attempt.

**Recovery:** Depends on which procedure is performed and what level of anesthesia (local or general) was utilized. Your partner should expect some soreness and perhaps some bruising; his surgeon can tell him specifically what to expect after his procedure. With all of these procedures—whether performed due to obstructive or nonobstructive azoospermia—ICSI will be used to achieve fertilization in order to ensure that all the hard work put into retrieving sperm is not wasted. Additionally, your physicians will want to cryopreserve (freeze) as much sperm as possible to ensure that you have future attempts at fertilization.

## Supporting the Infertile Man

As almost any woman knows, most men tend to internalize problems, withdraw, and become general pains in the asses when their manhood is questioned. Many men flat out refuse to have a semen analysis performed and refuse to acknowledge even the possibility that *they* could be the problem. The irony is that men are just as likely as women are to be the cause of infertility, and their workup is a lot less intensive. Thanks to ICSI, male-factor problems are generally easier to solve, too. And yet women bear the hardship of infertility a thousand times better than most men. Do I sound like a sexist? Well then, I guess I am.

But you have to live with him, and there's nothing worse than a withdrawn, uncommunicative partner, so let's talk about ways to help him cope. First understand that he (just like you) may have taken his fertility for granted. Machismo is completely tied up with ideas of fatherhood, so not being able to father a child makes your man feel less of a man. Add the possibility that he might not be able to carry on his family name or genes, and you've a situation that can be (and often is) emotionally overpowering. When I discovered that I probably wouldn't be able to carry a baby to term, I felt like less of a woman, even though I understood that the two things aren't related. So I don't underestimate how infuriating and gut-wrenching this can be for anyone.

Helping your husband get past his feelings of inadequacy can be even tougher when his infertility is related to sexual dysfunction. And sometimes feeling like less of a man can lead to sexual dysfunction. Some men dismiss their dysfunction by saying things like, "What's the point in getting it up if it ain't shootin' real bullets?" The whole sex-on-demand thing that comes with infertility doesn't help, either. It is bad enough when the zest has gone out of your sex life, but it's probably worse to continually "produce" into a little cup; especially when some stranger is on the other side of the wall waiting for his specimen, not to mention the wives pacing outside in the hallway. And while we're on the subject, *don't do this to your man!* Do him a favor, go wait in the waiting room, and leave him to do his business in the relative privacy the medical office has provided him. Trust me! He doesn't need to hear your heels *click, click, clicking* outside.

Infertility is hard enough on a marriage. Loss of physical intimacy can be deadly for some couples. So try to help your guy cope with this devastating news by trying to maintain your sex life. Try a romantic dinner (with a nice bottle of wine), a vacation in some luxe Caribbean resort (if you can still afford it), or maybe some soft porn. Whatever it is that might help put the romance or oomph back in your bed, give it a try. You need to stay physically close right now, even if you're not talking. If talking is getting to be a problem, too (are conversations about doing the dishes getting a little stressful for you? Hey, I've been there; tell me about it!), you may need to take a step back before you can move closer together again.

First, try to give him some space. You may be feeling alone, overwhelmed and stressed, but you need to tell your husband that you know he's having a really hard time accepting the diagnosis. It's okay if he doesn't want to talk about it now but tell him that eventually the two of you need to make some decisions together. Maybe plan a time together when you're in a neutral location (not at home, not at work, not at a doctor's office) to talk about it. Choosing someplace where you feel safe will help you to unburden. Take a drive somewhere, go for a long walk, or to your favorite restaurant. I know you're going to go nuts waiting for your conversation, so get busy researching treatment options. Cut out articles from magazines, newspapers, and even medical journals (if you're into that kinda thing) so you can tell him what you've discovered and direct him to source material if he wants to do his own reading. You'll feel proactive, and he'll (hopefully) feel a sense of relief at not having to talk about "it" for a while.

Second, you *must* stop nagging and criticizing him about the color of his tie or taking the garbage out. We all do this, and it's really horrible. There is more than one right way to do things. As a beloved wise woman once told me: There's more than one way to change a diaper. As long as it holds in the poop, who cares how it was done! You wanna get to the point where you're fighting over how to change a diaper? Leave him be! He feels horrible enough without you picking at him!

And speaking of feeling horrible, it might be a good idea to find ways to compliment him and boost his ego. Don't overdo it. Every now and again, just try to find a way to remind him about why you love him so much. He probably wonders if you'd rather divorce him and find a fertile partner right about now; a little love and a little praise will go a long way to helping him feel better about himself.

Once you've given him some time and space, you really do need to try to talk about your fertility and how it makes you both feel. Some men open up more easily than others. You may need to see the doctor together so you can both ask questions at the same time. You may want to seek help from your clergy person or rabbi, or consult a therapist who specializes in infertility-related issues. Or maybe you both can just sit down and make a list of pros and cons presented by your treatment options and see where it leads.

Whatever it takes, start talking. Honor your partner's conversational style, attitudes (he might be reluctant now to use donor sperm but not two days or two months from now), and his fears. Sometimes acknowledging your husband's or partner's feelings is all that's needed to make him feel better.

# Deciding Which Family-Building Option Is Best for You

## IT'S ALL A QUESTION OF NEEDLES

Now that you've subjected yourself to a battery of tests and feel like you've had, and have had, a zillion people looking at your private parts, it's time to make some decisions. What's next? All family-building options are equally valid. *No option should be considered last resort or second best.*

When Charlie and I first started our infertility treatment, I was adamant about not starting with IVF. I thought it was a treatment option for desperate, seriously, seriously infertile couples. I was *very wrong* about this, and I wasted almost a year with inseminations when, in fact, IVF was the best and fastest way for me to get pregnant. IVF is—and should be considered—a first-line treatment for many couples.

Similarly, I thought adoption was a concession of failure and that only couples with no other alternatives adopted. I realize I might have been a lot happier if I'd skipped IVF and started building my family through adoption right from the beginning. Adoption was my second choice (IVF came first), but it was by no means the second-*best* choice. Adoption was (is) right for me. I would've realized this sooner had I not been so closed off to it.

So this chapter is about having the right information when making decisions about treatment, and it's about having the right perspective about treatment and nontreatment options. Do not make the mistakes I did. Remove all the stupid labels, misguided characterizations, and antiquated notions about what is the *right way* to build a family, and you can avoid a lot of mistakes and delays. Let me tell you something: the only right way to build your family is the way *you decide* to do it. Got that? You, dear reader, rule!

No one other than you and your partner should decide how you'll build your family (except maybe your RE). You probably didn't ask other people when they thought it was time for you to have a baby, and you probably (I hope) didn't ask your brother-in-law with the five kids under six years of age what sex positions they used to conceive their babies. So why would you ask anyone (except a medical professional or clergy person) which path to parenthood is best for you? I'm going to discuss your options in a nonjudgmental format (alphabetical order) with all the pros and cons, expenses, and hassles involved in each; then you and your partner can make a game plan. And you should make a game plan; map out your journey before you begin, and establish preliminary timelines and alternatives for what you'll do if a treatment option fails. You can always revise your game plan as you go along, but it will be valuable as you move down your path.

As a needle-phobe, I can appreciate how concerned some women are about how much medical intervention—how many needles—is involved with each family-building option. Accordingly, I have provided a little needle symbol ( ), which will give you a quick sense of how much intervention each treatment involves. The fewer the needles next to a section, the less invasive that option is; the scale ranges from one (minimal medical stuff) to five needles (look out! we're talking high-tech stuff involved!). If there are no needles, that means there's no needly medical stuff involved at all (yippee!). Similarly, I've provided dollar signs to indicate how expensive a treatment option is ($). Each dollar sign signifies roughly $10,000 worth of expenses. Five dollar signs mean you're looking at major—as much as $50,000—financial outlays; no dollar sign means that you're looking at a "low-cost" treatment option that should cost less than $10,000. Now, I know, "low-cost" and less than $10,000 don't usually go together. One of the less pleasant aspects of infertility treatment and family building is that it's shockingly expensive. We'll talk about how to pay for it in chapter 9. Now, let's look at the different ways you can build your beautiful family.

## Adoption $$-$$$$

**What it is:** Adoption is a beautiful thing. It involves opening your heart and home to a child who may or may not look anything like you but desperately needs parents and love and nurturing. Adoption involves a leap of faith and a leap of love. There's no painful medical treatment connected with adoption, but there may be disappointment. Sometimes adoptions don't work the way we want them to or when we want them to. Sometimes birth mothers decide to parent their children; foreign countries sometimes suddenly close adoption programs weeks before you're scheduled to go pick up your child. But adoption is guaranteed. That's right, it's *guaranteed*. That is something no doctor can ever say about infertility treatment. You may need patience and fortitude, but in the end you will have a successful adoption.

Once you choose the type of adoption you want—domestic, international, agency, facilitator, or private attorney—and set the wheels in motion, the only way you won't get a baby is if you decide *not* to adopt. Yes, you'll have to jump through a lot of hoops (like getting your home study done, one of the state-approval requirements for adoption), but if your heart is open and you're ready to take the most incredible leap of love possible, you can save a lot of time and angst (and maybe even money) by choosing adoption rather than undergoing infertility treatment.

One of the few downsides to adoption is that you may have to give up some of your fantasies about how you become a mom. This is also true with infertility treatments like IVF, but adoption requires a larger adjustment. If IVF is successful, you get pregnant. If you're adopting, you get the baby without the belly (for some of you this may turn out to be a good thing). Even though you might know that your baby will be born in a matter of days, no one else will. Because you don't have that (big, stretch-mark-covered) belly, friends and family members may not think of you as "expecting," even though you are. Only truly enlightened friends (or those who've done some research, or known someone who's gone through the process of adoption) will think to throw you a baby shower. And you should have a baby shower!

Your experience will be different than most of your friends who are parents to be; they probably won't be able to relate to what you're going through. Talking to birth mothers or planning trips overseas may seem alien to your friends. They'll get used to it eventually, I promise. And your experience will be just as rewarding as theirs, if not more so.

Adoption is expensive. Insurance doesn't cover your expenses the way it does with medical treatment (although there is a newly burgeoning adoption insurance industry, which I'm skeptical about). There is a fairly substantial federal tax credit ($10,000 per adoption) that helps offset your costs and some companies even help employees pay for their adoption, but it will probably cost about $15,000 to adopt a baby. This is a realistic number; it's possible to spend less but not likely. And it's certainly possible to pay a lot more than that (we did). Infertility treatment is expensive, too, but you are more likely to have access to cost-deferring measures for infertility treatment than with adoption. I don't think any of this is fair.

Adoption shouldn't be treated differently than other family-building options; in fact, adoption should be encouraged. But it's not that way, at least not yet. The media is doing a great job of putting a modern face on adoption and dispelling common myths. The Hallmark Channel has an adoption show every week; Rosie O'Donnell, Oprah, and the *Today* show (just to name a few) have done specials on adoption. And thanks to people like Steven Spielberg (an adoptive dad several times over), there have been high-profile prime-time specials that educate people about adoption and encourage families to open their hearts to children and babies in need.

Adoption is a lot different today than it was even ten years ago. The days of registering with a state child-welfare agency and waiting four years (or more) for the phone to ring to find out there's a baby boy waiting for you somewhere are long gone. International adoptions, the Internet, and new ideas about semiopen and open adoption have created a whole new world of possibility for people who want to adopt. Waiting periods can be as short as six months or as long as two years. This is a big improvement! How long you will wait depends in part on what you're looking for out of the adoption experience.

**What's involved:** Let's start with *domestic adoptions*. Domestic adoption (in the U.S.) is usually the only way to adopt a newborn baby. You have two choices: you can work with an agency or a private attorney. Either way, if you want a newborn baby girl, delivered by an eighteen-year-old Caucasian girl who's never had a sip of alcohol (let alone tried an illegal drug), conceived the baby during her first act of intercourse, had prenatal care since the day she missed her period, and is living at home with her parents (one of whom happens to be a supportive, loving member of the clergy), well, you're in for a hell of a long wait. Don't get me wrong; if this is what you want, *go for it!* It will happen eventually, but you're going to have to be very patient because you might have to wait a pretty long time. If, however, you're open to a baby of unspecified gender from a birth mother who has a less than perfect background, your wait may be much shorter (maybe a year to eighteen months).

Increased flexibility on your part can shorten your wait even more. Are you Caucasian and open to adopting a Hispanic baby, open to a birth mother who has used drugs, smokes, or has issues with depression? These are questions only you and your partner can answer. But consider that most birth moms are in crisis and—like the rest of us—don't have ideal backgrounds. If you can accept birth mothers and birth fathers the way you accept family members facing a challenging situation, it will be a lot easier and faster to find a birth family.

Another question that factors in to how long you're going to wait: Are you open to "open adoption"? In the past, adoptions were completely closed. You didn't meet your child's biological parents and probably didn't get any medical history from them. This is no longer true in most adoptions. Now, it's much more common for birth parents and adoptive families to have contact. The degree of anonymity and contact maintained between the birth and adoptive families—before and after placement of the baby—distinguishes open and semiopen adoptions.

In both types of adoption, birth parents usually select the adoptive parents based on photos or a letter. This matching process can take place at any time during a birth mother's pregnancy. After the birth parents have chosen an adoptive family, the adoptive parents usually have an opportunity to review abbreviated medical and life histories and/or talk to the birth parents. The adoptive parents then choose whether they wish to adopt the baby or continue to search for another birth family. Here the similarities between semiopen and open adoption end.

In a semiopen adoption, there is a greater degree of anonymity maintained by the adoptive and birth families. While the two families may speak or even meet, often they only share their first names. Once the baby is placed for adoption, the adoptive parents may send cards or letters for a short (predetermined) period of time to let the birth parents know that the baby is healthy and happy. Some birth parents write a letter for their child to read later, to help explain why she was placed for adoption; some birth parents may even agree to meet their birth child later in life. But after this period of time has elapsed, the birth and adoptive families have no further contact.

In an open adoption, the adoptive parents and birth parents have a chance to get to know each other and to develop a long-term relationship. In a truly open adoption, the relationship between birth and adoptive parents doesn't end. Essentially, the two families unite and form a lifelong relationship. This is very scary to some adoptive families as it raises questions about authenticity (who is the authentic parent of the adopted child?) and fears that the birth parents may one day steal the child back. But this doesn't happen; the reality is that open adoptions are so successful that the families involved can't imagine having done it any other way.

An agency or private attorney can help you with a closed, semiopen, or open adoption. Agency adoptions may involve less risk than private adoptions using an attorney; fewer birth mothers choose to parent when agencies are involved. This may have something to do with the fact that agencies provide support and counseling for birth mothers/families. Whatever type of adoption you choose, expect and prepare for two things: First, you probably will have to speak with at least one birth mother over the phone before she will agree to place her baby with you (your attorney or agency can help educate you about how to talk to birth mothers, but let me tell you now, it's a very weird experience). Second, there is *always* a risk that the birth mother will decide to parent her baby. The circumstances under which a birth mother can decide to parent vary from state to state. Some states give birth mothers weeks or months to change their mind, while other states provide only a few hours.

It is more common for a birth mom to decide to parent before delivery but it can—and does—happen after birth. I've had two birth mothers decide to parent, each time after the baby was born. If this concerns you, talk to your agency or attorney and work only in states that have strict relinquishment laws. Our son's birth mother decided to parent him the day after he was born. My baby came home, but it took almost six months (an *unusually* long period of time) before his birth mom relinquished her parental rights. Our second adoption did not end as well; we wound up having to return the baby (a boy) three days after we took him home. Though each of these experiences was gut wrenching, I remain a huge adoption advocate.

Birth fathers can present issues, too, especially those who don't support the adoption plan or whose identity is unknown. Again, laws pertaining to consent vary from state to state. Reputable agencies and private attorneys can help you navigate these complex waters.

The decision to proceed with an attorney or agency will probably depend on cost and the level of risk you're willing to take. Some agencies are very expensive (the cost is usually determined on a sliding scale based on income), but the agency will do absolutely everything including screening potential birth mothers for you. They also handle legal issues and will see you through the process for one flat fee. Other agencies are less expensive and present financial options similar to those offered by private attorneys, who usually offer pay-as-you-go type systems. You'll pay your attorney a retainer (or the agency a fee), then pay for advertising and other marketing techniques. When a birth mother selects you, you'll probably pay for her medical and living expenses. If the birth mother chooses to parent, you may be out the money you paid her (although sometimes monies paid for living and medical expenses are placed in escrow and are partially refundable). Either way there are risks and advantages. If the first birth mother you agree to work with at an agency successfully places her baby with you, you may have paid more than you would've had you worked with a private attorney. But you may have done less work—looking for a birth mother can become a full-time job when you're doing a private adoption—and suffered fewer headaches.

Private adoptions often offer much more flexibility and independence and often impose fewer restrictions about the age, religion, and marital status of the adoptive parents than do agencies. Do the research to find the right agency or attorney for your needs. Some agencies are very flexible and some aren't. Some agencies offer a fee-for-service system instead of a flat fee, and some private attorneys might agree to accept a one-time fee up front.

If you choose to pursue an *international* adoption, you can work with either an agency or a facilitator (sometimes an attorney, sometimes not). And you've got many countries to choose from. Depending on the country you select, you can usually adopt a baby as young as seven weeks old. Some countries offer discounts to people who adopt two children. Most of the time you will need to make at least one trip to the country of your child's origin (sometimes two or even three trips will be required); although some programs will bring the baby to you in the United States.

International adoptions tend to be less expensive than domestic adoptions. But when you factor in the traveling expenses, they are still costly. International adoption also tends to be easier for older couples (those in their fifties) or same-sex couples or single parents. Some countries will only work with facilitators and not agencies, and accept only cash payments (this is a perfectly legal adoption). If you're squeamish about traveling with tens of thousands of dollars in cash, make sure you know what's expected before you decide what country, agency, or facilitator you're going to use.

*Foster care adoption* is another option. For those willing to risk a little heartbreak, this can be a wonderful way to adopt a baby or child. With foster care adoption, you register with your state to become foster parents. Once licensed, you will be contacted when there is a baby or child in need of a temporary home. Many of these babies or children will later become available for adoption. I have read many heartwarming stories about foster-adopt parents who've adopted newborns and children this way. If you're open to the concept, it may present a faster way to adopt a newborn than a private or agency-assisted domestic adoption. It's also a wonderful way to adopt an older child (most of whom are considered unadoptable). But there are risks; these babies and children *often* go back to their birth families. Make sure you're ready to be *foster* parents before you consider being a *foster-adoptive* parent.

There are a lot of agencies and facilitators you can use for international and domestic adoptions, and many of them aren't reputable. There are fewer agencies that specialize in domestic adoptions, but there are many more attorneys who claim to be adoption attorneys and will gladly take your money and waste your time. And even some of the agencies are scary. Be a thorough, well-educated consumer. Get recommendations from friends, family, medical professionals, clergy, RESOLVE, or AIA, and do your research. Attend seminars on adoption, talk to families who've adopted, read books and magazines (see the Resources section). Choose wisely and chose well, and you're more likely to have a satisfying, joy-filled adoption experience.

## Alternative Therapies

**What it is:** Many women and couples choose to completely bypass conventional medical treatment, opting instead to use alternative therapies. And there are those—like me—who use alternative therapies to complement conventional medical treatment. If you're interested in pursuing a holistic approach to infertility treatment, you've got several options. Homeopaths, naturopaths, acupuncture, mind-body work, hypnosis, diet, and meditation—when used alone or in combination—can be very effective.

**What's involved:** Acupuncture has recently gotten the attention of doctors, including reproductive endocrinologists! The theory behind acupuncture (in oversimplified terms) is that we're all made up of energy, and there are specific points or meridians of energy running along the body. If energy, chi, is blocked or doesn't flow freely though these meridians (areas of the body), then illness and disease—including infertility—result. Stimulating areas of the body with needles restores the energy flow to create harmony in the body and resolve illness.

One study published in a major reproductive medicine journal found that women who underwent acupuncture in combination with IVF had higher pregnancy rates than those who did not. The study recommended that acupuncture be more fully explored as an option for infertility treatment. Whether you choose to use only acupuncture or use it in combination with more conventional approaches to infertility treatment, acupuncture is a promising low-tech option. And don't be afraid of the needles; even a major needle-phobe like me can handle it!

Mind-body work also can also be an effective way to address infertility without medical treatment. Dr. Alice Domar has been doing groundbreaking work on the connection between mind and body in infertility. She has consistently found that women who meditate and use other stress-reduction and biofeedback techniques have higher conception rates. Contact information for Dr. Domar and other clinics with similar programs are listed in the Resources section if you want more information.

Changing your diet or consulting a naturopath or homeopath may also help restore balance and health in the body and facilitate pregnancy. Less tested than acupuncture and mind-body work, these holistic/lifestyle options have yielded results for many women. Naturopathic treatment for infertility aims to balance the hormone system through diet and moderate exercise. Homeopathy treats the entire person (mind and body) with herbal remedies and tries to harness the body's self-healing powers to correct conditions and imbalances that can cause infertility. Homeopathy, a popular and widely accepted form of medical treatment in Europe, is becoming more popular in the United States. But to date, there are no studies proving that homeopathy and naturopathy are effective ways to achieve pregnancy.

I explored many holistic alternatives when I was trying to become pregnant. I changed my diet to help treat my endometriosis; my symptoms diminished, and I had a better response to IVF drugs. Acupuncture helped me manage stress and other side effects of the IVF meds. I encourage you to consider alternative treatments as an adjunct to conventional treatment (remember to discuss all alternative therapies with your RE before you start) or as a complete alternative. I've listed some books in the Resources section that will help you learn more about these treatments.

## Child-Free Living

**What it is:** Living child-free is a frightening thought for many people. Usually, those who undergo fertility treatment want children desperately. Most infertile couples find they have a lot of grieving to go through before they can truly accept this idea of living without children. The loss of the image of themselves as mother and father and as a family unit is overpowering. This also isn't a lifestyle choice that's readily accepted in the United States. For many infertile couples, societal pressure can be an overwhelming obstacle to a child-free life.

Difficult though this decision is, there are many advantages. For couples with high-powered careers, there is no guilt or pressure to be home with children, no struggle over day care, no conflict between work and family. Travel and social life can be enjoyed spontaneously, often at a whim. Financial pressure is reduced when you don't have to worry about how to pay for college or day care. You can enjoy other people's children without the drain of sleep-deprived nights, tantrums, and adolescent angst.

**What's involved:** If child-free living is something you and your partner are considering, make sure you both want to pursue this path together. If there is conflict or concern over the choice, seek counseling. Take time with the decision; explore the lifestyle before deciding whether it's right for you. It may take some time before you've healed emotionally and can fully experience the benefits of a child-free life. Remember, this is not an irreversible decision. If you eventually decide against a child-free life, you still have options for building your family. Nothing is forever unless you want it to be.

## Egg and Sperm Donation $

**What it is:** Some types of infertility preclude the use of your genetic material to achieve pregnancy. For these people, ovum and sperm donation offer wonderful options for achieving pregnancy. For women with poor ovarian response, poor fertilization results, who've failed to achieve a pregnancy after repeated IVF attempts or have genetic issues and a high likelihood of miscarriage, egg donation offers exceptional pregnancy rates. Women who use donated eggs have pregnancy rates comparable to those of young women with no fertility problems. Similarly, sperm donation offers a wonderful option for parenthood to men who have untreatable infertility or don't wish to use high-tech procedures like ICSI or surgical sperm retrieval techniques.

**What's involved:** Because most people don't want to lose the opportunity to have a genetic link to their child, choosing egg or sperm donation can be tough. There are other emotional complexities as well. For example, do you tell your child that she is the product of a donor's egg? Or do you keep it a secret? Many people argue against maintaining secrecy, but it's a highly individual choice. There is absolutely no shame in choosing this option for building your family so—theoretically—there should be no shame in sharing this information with your child or other family members. And if your child later discovers the facts surrounding her conception, there may be a lot of hurt and anger to resolve.

If you choose egg and/or sperm donation, you'll probably select a donor from an anonymous profile provided by your clinic or sperm bank. Your clinic will prescreen donors for characteristics such as height, weight, hair and eye color, and any educational or religious preferences you may express. You then get an opportunity to review the donor's profile before deciding whether or not to proceed.

There also is a growing trend in ovum donation in which you contract with an independent agency (not your clinic) to select and *meet* your donor. Another option is to have a sister, brother, or other friend or relative contribute the egg or sperm. However, the lack of anonymity involved concerns many couples. If you choose an open ovum donation, you're facing issues similar to those with open adoption. There is a complex personal connection when you know your ovum donor. Legally, however, (at least to date) the donor has no legal rights with respect to the child (as opposed to a birth mother in an adoption or a more traditional surrogacy). Agencies that offer open ovum donation will make sure there is a binding legal contract to govern your relationship.

Ovum donors are usually young women who've been thoroughly screened for any genetic condition or illness that could impair the quality of her eggs or be transmitted to an embryo. The risk of miscarriage and genetic problems (younger women's eggs have fewer chromosomal problems) is extremely low. Indeed, women over forty who undergo IVF egg donation don't have amniocentesis. Sperm donors are also thoroughly screened, and the more reputable sperm banks require donors to undergo infectious disease testing.

The donor recipients—especially female recipients—are also thoroughly screened to ensure a high likelihood for a resulting pregnancy. This may mean that you undergo a mock cycle to see how your body responds to the medications used to prepare your uterus to receive an embryo. Some fertility centers also require you to undergo counseling to ensure that any psychological issues presented by ovum donation have been adequately resolved and that you're psychologically prepared for issues that may arise later in your child's life.

Depending on your reproductive condition, egg and sperm donation can be a low-tech, low-cost approach to building your family. If male-factor infertility is your sole impediment to pregnancy, a natural cycle IUI using donor sperm (IUI cycles are discussed in greater detail later in this chapter and again in chapters 11 and 12) may get you pregnant. If you've got female-factor infertility on top of male-factor, you might try a medicated cycle of IUI using donor sperm (more needles, more money), or you might consider IVF (even more needles and, of course, more money). With ovum donation, you'll have to undergo an IVF cycle that will be timed with that of your donor. You won't undergo surgical egg retrieval, but you will have an embryo transfer (see chapter 12), which means needles and lots of money. However, both egg and sperm donation tend to result in very good pregnancy rates, so you may not need many attempts before you achieve pregnancy.

Some clinics allow ovum donors to share their eggs with two or more recipient families, which can reduce the cost to each recipient. If you're comfortable knowing your donor likely will be creating half-siblings for any offspring you conceive during your cycle, this may be a great cost-saving option for you. If, however, this makes you uncomfortable, you have the option of using all your donor eggs and paying full price. Seriously consider freezing any embryos you don't use on your first transfer, thus maximizing the money you've spent and your chances for conceiving again. These frozen embryos can be used later if your first transfer doesn't result in a live birth or to create a sibling at a later point in time. You'll need to discuss these options (sharing the donor's eggs and freezing embryos) with your clinic before undergoing a donor egg cycle.

When considering egg and sperm donation, be sure to balance the stress of potential multiple failed cycles using your own genetic material against the need to get on with life and pregnancy. Age usually plays a big role in the decision to undergo an IVF egg donor cycle; if you're forty-three, you've probably got better odds at getting pregnant using donor eggs than your own. Only you can decide whether you'd rather be pregnant in the next few months (but without a complete genetic link to your child) or whether you should try a few cycles using your own genetic material, even if it means more time and a higher emotional and financial cost. Sometimes the right option is the middle road, to try one or two cycles without donor material, and if that fails, move on to a donor cycle.

## Embryo Donation 💉💉 $

**What it is:** Embryo donation offers a newer option for building a family. Instead of adopting a newborn, young infant, or child, you are using another couple's embryo to attempt a pregnancy (How cool is that?) The embryo is transferred to your uterus after you undergo treatment to optimize your uterine environment for implantation (the same as for egg donation). These embryos often come from couples who have achieved the family they dreamed of through IVF and don't wish to have more children. Left with frozen embryos that they don't wish to use, many couples offer to donate these embryos instead of having them destroyed or used for research. However, many embryos that families wish to donate are deemed unsuitable, often due to the female donor's age, her history of previous pregnancy loss, or other medical factors.

**What's involved:** Most embryo donations are closed and are handled in much the same manner as egg or sperm donation. However, due to moral complexities (you've got two married donors and full siblings) there are additional hurdles to deal with. Initially, you and your husband are matched with the embryo donors based on physical characteristics. Both couples go through infectious disease screening and counseling (any program that doesn't provide or recommend counseling for couples considering embryo donation should be considered less than ideal). Once a match is made, you'll be presented with complex legal documents. It is a good idea to hire a good family lawyer, experienced with embryo donation, to review these documents (you can contact RESOLVE, the AIA, or ASRM for a referral).

Embryo donation hasn't been thoroughly tested by courts. Each state has its own laws, so make sure that the state in which you live, the state in which the embryo transfer will take place, and the state where the biological parents live will enforce the agreements you enter into. The American Society for Reproductive Medicine has set forth legal and ethical standards that it recommends before embryo donation is entered into. You may want to review these standards with your attorney.

I think this is a wonderful option for building a family, provided you're comfortable knowing that your child has full siblings out there somewhere and that certain of the issues adopted children face (identity issues and reuniting with birth families to name two) may be more intense and complex (questions like how come I wound up frozen and not my siblings?). I have listed some additional source material for learning about embryo donation in the Resources section.

## Intrauterine Insemination 💉💉 $

**What it is:** Intrauterine insemination (IUI) is a fairly low-tech, inexpensive option for treating certain kinds of infertility. More good news: most insurance plans pay for it (New York State just mandated coverage for IUIs, whereas it won't require insurance companies to pay for IVF)! Once your eggs have developed (see chapters 10 and 11 for more info), your partner's (or a donor's) sperm is placed in your uterus using a small catheter inserted into your uterus through your cervix (usually painless). Everything is timed so that the sperm enters your uterus as you're about to ovulate. By getting the sperm into just the right place at just the right time, egg and sperm have the best possible chance of meeting and conceiving your baby.

**A word to the wise:** | If you've got a doctor who's letting you do medicated IUIs with no end in sight (I've heard of women doing ten or more IUIs), find a new RE. You're wasting time and money when there are better, more effective ways of getting you pregnant.

**What's involved:** There are two types of IUIs: natural IUI cycles and those that use medication to stimulate multiple egg production. Most women who undergo IUI take medication. But no surgical procedures or extended recuperation periods are involved. And IUI usually doesn't involve too many needles (always a good thing, yes?); sometimes IUIs are performed using an ingestible medication (Clomid) instead of the stronger injectable meds used during IVF.

IUIs usually are recommended as a first step in infertility treatment, especially for those who don't have insurance or are hesitant about undergoing IVF. But IUI isn't always the best step. Some types of infertility can be treated very effectively using IUI; however, many types of infertility are treated more successfully and faster using IVF (endometriosis and male factor infertility that may require ICSI). Many couples start their infertility treatment with IUI, fail to get pregnant, and then move on to IVF and immediately get pregnant.

If you've decided you're only going to allocate a certain amount of time, effort, or money to treating your infertility, IUI may not be the best or fastest way to conceive. If, however, you have insurance coverage (or tons of money) and have decided that if IUI fails, you're willing to continue with other treatments (and pull out the bigger guns), then it makes a lot of sense to start with IUIs. If you get pregnant with IUI, you've saved yourself the emotional and physical expenses associated with more invasive treatments like IVF. If IUI isn't successful, you know you're plodding along on the path and still have a great chance of conceiving with IVF.

But please be aware: my last—and perhaps most important—comment about IUI is that statistically, if you're going to conceive this way, you will do so within the first *four* attempts. If you start with IUI (as I did), set a limit for the number of assisted cycles (those using drugs to stimulate your ovaries to produce more eggs) you're willing to undertake and have a plan for what treatment options, if any, you will pursue if IUI fails.

## In Vitro Fertilization 💉💉💉💉 $-$$

**What it is:** In vitro fertilization is truly amazing and miraculous. It's also scary as hell. Mostly this has to do with the misguided preconceptions most women have about IVF (like my silly misconception that only desperate couples do IVF). Also, the process is very intensive. Most people do what I did. They start first with IUI, are extremely frustrated when it fails, and move on to IVF, often with little or no emotional resources left to help them cope with the grueling process. Remember that I said treating infertility is a *process*, but there are certain decisions you could make that would *speed up* the process? Here's one of them. Choosing IVF first over other treatment options may be the smartest thing you can do for yourself. It's certainly a tough path, but it may be the most effective.

Current statistics consistently show that 75 percent of couples (including those who failed to conceive with IUI) conceive within their first three or four attempts at IVF. For many couples, IUI is a less intimidating and less expensive treatment option, whereas IVF is often a faster, more direct route to pregnancy. The fact that your insurance company likely will pay for only a certain type of treatment or limits the total amount you can spend on treatment (not enough to pay for one complete IVF cycle but enough to pay for a couple of IUI cycles) only adds to your confusion. IVF *is* expensive (heck, I racked up $85,000 in IVF charges, only some of which were covered by insurance) but I think we let fear of IVF interfere with logic. I sure as hell did.

Your fourth IUI may be successful, but what about the emotional toll it takes to get through six months or more of treatment with IUI, when you might well have gotten pregnant on your first IVF cycle in about two months? Factor in your frustration level as you start IVF after IUI failed, and you're now asking yourself to face your fear of IVF, undergo more intense treatment, and spend more money when you're exhausted, depressed, and perhaps rapidly running out of insurance money (if you're not contemplating taking serious mood altering drugs at this point you're *way* ahead of the game; most of us would kill for some Valium and Zoloft). Putting aside questions of how best to deal with insurance issues (see chapter 9), if you do IVF, you need to be mentally strong. Let me demystify IVF a little bit so you can—at least—make a more informed decision than I did.

**What it is:** Let's talk about what IVF is (and isn't). IVF is *not* only for desperate people with major infertility problems. Choosing IVF does *not* mean that all hope is lost. IVF relies on sophisticated technology and creates the greatest likelihood of conception possible in any one cycle. More aspects of human conception are controlled and monitored with IVF than with any other method of achieving pregnancy. For most couples undergoing IVF in a state-of-the-art facility, IVF gives them odds of conceiving in any one cycle that are three or sometimes four times higher than that of your average fertile twenty-five-year-old couple (who've got roughly a 20 percent chance of conceiving in any one menstrual cycle). IVF (in a good clinic) routinely offers success (pregnancy/conception) rates near 50 to 60 percent per cycle. Advanced coculture programs and blastocyst transfer increase success rates to 80 percent per cycle in some clinics.

During IVF, doctors use medication to help you produce the best possible quality eggs, surgically remove them from your ovaries in a minimally invasive outpatient procedure, and then combine them with your partner's sperm, watch for fertilization and embryo growth, and then transfer (on average) three healthy embryos to your uterus where, hopefully, they'll implant and grow. The first advantage to IVF is that you don't need your fallopian tubes to achieve conception (as you do with old-fashioned conception, IUI, GIFT, and ZIFT) so women with tubes damaged by endo or other disease have a great chance at conception. IVF offers other benefits as well. This process is diagnostic because your doctor can (1) see what your eggs look like, (2) see how fertilization takes place, and (3) see how the embryos grow. Each of these steps can reveal a great deal about why you aren't achieving pregnancy and at the same time help you get pregnant.

Sometimes the embryologist discovers that the sperm cannot penetrate the egg to achieve fertilization. This could be because the zona pellucida (the shell) of the egg is too brittle, so the sperm cannot penetrate the egg. This only can be detected with microscopes and by experienced embryologists (the people who take care of your eggs and embryos). Techniques like ICSI (see chapter 6) can help IVF patients achieve fertilization when the sperm cannot penetrate the egg.

Sometimes egg and sperm look completely normal, but your embryos aren't healthy and don't grow well. Sometimes this can be corrected with special culture mediums (the nutrient-rich substance that fertilized eggs are put in to help them grow). Some clinics have state-of-the-art coculture programs that use your endometrial tissue (it's cloned and grown in the lab) or your blood, which when mixed with standard culture medium, provides a better environment in which poor quality embryos may grow. After your first cycle, your RE may discover that you could benefit from an advanced coculture program in a subsequent cycle. These are only a few of the otherwise "undetectable" problems preventing pregnancy that can be observed—and diagnosed—during IVF.

IVF is a physically grueling process. Many women who achieve pregnancy with IVF from their first cycle say it was a breeze (I think it's like childbirth; you forget the pain when you get the baby), but there are just as many women who refuse to do it more than once no matter *what*.

**What's Involved:** I talk in great detail about IVF cycles in chapters 11 and 12, so I'm just going to share the bottom line here. IVF means injecting yourself with medication (or having someone you love inject you) in your lower abdomen or thigh at least once a day (if not two or three times a day), having many uncomfortable ultrasounds (sometimes while you're gushing blood), two minor surgical procedures (is there really such a thing as minor surgery?), being strung out on hormones (remember Charlie's nickname for me on stims? RLB, or raving lunatic bitch), on bed rest (for the first time, bed rest isn't fun), afraid to sneeze or poop (God forbid you do something to jiggle those embryos!), and absolutely petrified that it didn't work (now you really need that Valium).

Each woman reacts differently, but there's no doubt that almost every woman who undergoes IVF later admits that it was extremely difficult (and those who don't are either in massive denial or are *lying* to you). While I was going through IVF, I thought it was manageable, doable, and livable. When I stopped IVF and got my life back, I realized just how demanding it was. I had *nightmares* about injections for months. If you choose this route, do not underestimate how much support you will need. Even if you get pregnant right away, that one cycle will challenge you in more ways than you can comprehend.

Trust me, no matter how prepared you think you are for IVF, or how many people you know who've gone through it, or how much research you've done, or how strong you think you are, you've *never* faced a demon like this. When you get through your first IVF cycle, you achieve a special status; you're the most devoted, committed, and focused of all future mothers. Your kids are truly walking into strong and loving arms and are truly, truly wanted and blessed, or you wouldn't have worked so hard to get them.

So now you know. IVF is perhaps the fastest route to pregnancy, but it's also probably the hardest.

## GIFT (Gamete Intrafallopian Transfer)
💉💉💉💉💉 $$

**What it is:** GIFT is a variation on IVF in which fertilization takes place inside the woman's body instead of in a laboratory. The eggs are surgically removed and placed inside the fallopian tube with the sperm *before* fertilization takes place. Only women with at least one undamaged fallopian tube are candidates for this treatment. Originally GIFT was a good choice for couples with unexplained infertility, endometriosis, mild male factor infertility, cervical problems, luteinized unruptured follicle syndrome, or where it was necessary to ensure that the sperm reached the fallopian tube. GIFT also has been an option for some couples whose religion does not permit IVF. Catholicism, for example, forbids the use of certain assisted reproductive technologies used during IVF.

Recent advancements in IVF technology, however, have made GIFT obsolete. If GIFT fails to get you pregnant, you don't know whether the failure was due to lack of fertilization or something else. One of the major benefits of IVF is that doctors can see whether fertilization has taken place and how well the embryo is growing. For those cases where sperm are not capable of fertilizing an egg, with IVF, fertilization can be assisted using ICSI. Also, GIFT requires a laparoscopy, a much more invasive surgical procedure than is performed during IVF. And recent advancements in culture medium (the stuff embryos are placed in to nourish them and help them grow) and coculture programs during IVF have further increased fertilization rates. In the early days of IVF and GIFT, GIFT was preferred because sperm and egg were placed in the most ideal environment in which embryos could develop; the culture medium then used for IVF wasn't as conducive to embryo growth as the nutrient rich fallopian tube. But now that the medium used to culture (grow) embryos outside the fallopian tube has been improved, IVF fertilization and pregnancy rates routinely exceed those of GIFT. Finally, the ability to culture embryos to the more evolved blastocyst stage (see chapter 12), results in higher pregnancy rates and lower multiple birth rates. Because physicians prefer to minimize risk of multiple births, IVF and/or blastocyst transfer is preferable to GIFT as it decreases the risk of high order multiple conception (triplets or greater). Unless there is a religious objection, most couples will be counseled to use IVF.

**What's involved:** The woman undergoes an IVF cycle in which she is stimulated to produce a large number of eggs (same old, same old). The eggs are surgically removed from her ovaries (same old, same old) and are mixed with her partner's sperm (same old, same old). This is where similarity with IVF ends. At the time the sperm and eggs (the gametes) are mixed, they're surgically (during a laparoscopy) returned to the woman's fallopian tubes where, if all goes well, fertilization takes place.

## Natural Cycle IVF 💉 $

**What it is:** Natural cycle IVF is a cycle without any medication to stimulate the ovaries to produce eggs. You will rely instead on the natural ovulatory cycle to produce an egg. The idea is that some women with poor ovarian response seem to produce poorer quality eggs and embryos during a stimulated IVF cycle (one using medication) than in cycles without medication (go figure!). In the hope that one healthier egg will make a healthy embryo when three or four unhealthy eggs may not make any healthy embryos, REs hope natural cycle IVF will help these women achieve pregnancy. Natural cycle IVF is also gaining popularity as a lower-tech, lower-cost option for achieving pregnancy for couples who need ICSI or for those at high risk for conceiving a high-order multiple birth (usually very young couples).

Research on natural cycle IVF is still developing. It seems to work well for certain couples. It is definitely lower-tech and less expensive, but it may not give every couple as great odds at conception as conventional IVF. If you're interested in natural cycle IVF, you should discuss the pros and cons with your RE.

**What's involved:** Patients are monitored for ovulation (using blood work and ultrasound) and when they're ready to ovulate, the egg(s) is surgically removed (the same egg retrieval procedure used for conventional IVF) and combined with sperm to achieve fertilization. If the resulting embryo(s) is healthy, it's returned to the uterus (again the same procedure used during IVF).

## Preimplantation Genetic Diagnosis (PGD) $

**What it is:** Preimplantation genetic diagnosis isn't exactly a treatment for infertility; it's more of a diagnostic tool used in conjunction with IVF. Many people don't know about it but could benefit from it. PGD enables doctors to screen embryos created during an IVF cycle so they can ensure that only genetically healthy embryos are transferred back to the uterus. Centers that perform PGD recommend it for women over thirty-seven or thirty-eight years of age, those with prior miscarriages due to a chromosomal error, multiple unexplained pregnancy losses, repeated IVF failures, or who have a genetic condition, translocation, or other chromosomal error.

For some unknown reason, embryos created during IVF have more chromosomal anomalies than scientists expected. Chromosomal problems can lead to early embryo death or miscarriage. "Advanced maternal age" often results in eggs with chromosomal damage. Doctors are also finding that men with male-factor problems may also be more likely to produce genetically damaged sperm (even those sperm that appear normal may be genetically impaired). Random chromosomal accidents, translocated genes (genes that are misplaced on the DNA strand), or too many or too few chromosomes can all contribute to premature embryo death.

**What's involved:** PGD checks the genetic composition of your embryos before they're transferred to your uterus. PGD was developed to help couples with inheritable genetic problems, doctors remove one or two of the cells of an embryo on the third day of its life (the cells are called blastomeres) and analyze their genetic composition to determine whether that embryo contains inheritable diseases (like Tay-Sachs disease, cystic fibrosis, thalassemia, sickle cell anemia, hemophilia, muscular dystrophy, and spinal muscular atrophy) or other chromosomal problems that may result in that child contracting the disease/illness. PGD can also determine the gender of the embryo, but virtually every lab in the United States that performs PGD *refuses* to preselect embryos based on gender, unless you or your husband carry an inheritable disease that afflicts a particular gender. PGD now also is used to help couples who may have other genetic issues that result in IVF failure or miscarriage.

While PGD reduces miscarriage rates and is successful at screening embryos that carry diseases like Tay-Sachs, there are some things that you should know about PGD. First, it doesn't always work to identify chromosomally impaired embryos, and it cannot yet test for all kinds of chromosomes. Patients who utilize PGD are still advised to undergo amniocentesis, chorionic villous sampling, or other prenatal tests. And PGD comes with risk. Sometimes—even with extremely skilled technicians—an embryo doesn't survive the process of having a blastomere removed and will arrest (die) after PGD has been performed.

If you're contemplating PGD, it's imperative that you select an established facility with high PGD success rates. Contact the American Society for Reproductive Medicine, RESOLVE, or AIA for a referral. If you've suffered multiple miscarriages, IVF failure, or carry an inheritable disease, PGD offers hope for the family you've always dreamed of. It will add to the cost of your IVF procedure (it usually costs about $2,500), but the money may well be worth the peace of mind and added chance of achieving a successful pregnancy and healthy child.

## Surrogates and Gestational Care 👶👶👶 $$$$$

**What it is:** In vitro fertilization surrogacy, also known as gestational surrogacy, provides a host uterus for a couple's embryo. A woman who is unable to carry a pregnancy to term but is able to create embryos with IVF can contract with another woman to carry the pregnancy. This surrogate merely provides a uterus in which the embryo grows and develops. She has no biological connection to the embryo. Traditional surrogacy is different in that the surrogate donates her egg and her uterus to the infertile couple to help them achieve a pregnancy.

These two forms of third-party parenting may sound scary to infertile couples. Everyone has heard of at least one horror story about a surrogate who refused to relinquish parental rights to a baby she'd agreed to carry for another couple. Legal protections, however, are now in place to protect would-be parents against this kind of trouble. Most states have specific laws that govern surrogacy relationships. Some make it illegal for anyone other than an unpaid friend or relative to carry a couple's child; other states are far more permissive and allow couples to contract with third parties to provide a host uterus or an egg and uterus to an infertile couple. Many fertility centers can recommend ways to minimize legal risks. Counseling and screening by fertility clinics and agencies that specialize in third-party surrogate arrangements (yes, believe it or not, there are agencies that do nothing but help you find a suitable surrogate) can offer further protection.

**What's involved:** Surrogates and gestational carriers are evaluated—both medically and psychologically—to ensure that only the healthiest, most stable women participate in this process. Additionally, thanks to advancements in reproductive science, traditional surrogacy (involving a third party donating an egg and providing a uterus) no longer requires the biological father to have intercourse with the third-party donor. Today, most surrogates conceive through insemination or IVF techniques.

Surrogacy is phenomenally expensive (even I—spender of insane amounts of money to build my family—shudder at the cost). When using an agency to facilitate the arrangement, the average cost for a gestational carrier is $50,000 to $80,000. This includes the costs incurred by the surrogate, the costs of IVF, and the agency's costs. You can reduce the amount somewhat (by about $20,000) by locating your own surrogate and hiring a private attorney to structure your relationship and obligations. However, there are greater risks involved. A far greater percentage of independent surrogate arrangements end in discord without a resulting pregnancy. Most physicians and attorneys do not recommend undertaking an independent arrangement unless it involves a family member.

Traditional surrogacy is somewhat less expensive, $30,000 to $50,000 on average, including medical, legal, and agency costs. The reduced cost derives largely from the fact that usually the surrogate doesn't undergo expensive IVF procedures (instead relying on IUI) in order to get pregnant.

Third-party parenting provides hope to seemingly hopeless couples. After my multiple miscarriages, Charlie and I seriously discussed using a gestational carrier. For personal and financial reasons, we chose adoption; but I don't rule out the possibility of gestational surrogacy in the future.

Surrogacy is an intensely personal decision. It's hard enough to accept the fact that you can't carry a baby to term; it may be even harder to watch someone else carry your baby for you. However, with proper counseling and professional help, surrogacy is a good and increasingly popular way to build a family.

## ZIFT (Zygote Intrafallopian Transfer)
$$

**What it is:** A variation on GIFT (see above), ZIFT enables doctors to replace fertilized eggs (zygotes) to a woman's fallopian tubes. ZIFT is outdated and outmoded, and it's hard to find a facility that still performs this treatment. I doubt that a good RE will recommend ZIFT to you (and if she does, you might want to consider finding out why and maybe even find a new RE). Most IVF programs today offer higher pregnancy rates with fewer surgical interventions and greater chance of preventing high-order multiple births.

**What's involved:** As with GIFT and IVF, the woman undergoes a stimulation protocol that causes her to produce a large number of eggs. The eggs are surgically removed and then fertilized (ICSI can be used to achieve fertilization). Twenty-four hours later, the woman undergoes a laparoscopy during which the fertilized eggs (zygotes) are returned to her fallopian tubes with the hope that they will successfully make their way to the woman's uterus and implant. As with GIFT, only women with at least one functioning fallopian tube are candidates for this treatment.

## Other Things to Consider When Choosing Infertility Treatment

There are a few more things you need to know about the treatment-based options (like IUI and IVF) before you can make a fully informed decision about which is right for you and your partner. The first is the risk of *multiple birth*. Many women I know, myself included, don't think much about this when facing IUI, IVF, or third-party parenting arrangements. Our attitude is something like "get me pregnant first; I'll worry about triplets and quadruplets later!" Yeah right. You *need* to worry about this now before you're hopped up on hormones and have been pinched by needles, poked, prodded, anesthetized, and otherwise manipulated beyond the bounds of normal human comprehension.

Multiple birth is a very real risk, and there are many physicians who push the boundaries of safety in order to maximize their success rates. While transferring four or five embryos or stimulating you in an IUI cycle to produce five or six follicles might enhance your clinic's success rates, it also puts you in the unenviable position of having to choose between your health and that of your babies. Multiple births—even when properly and expertly managed—result in lower-birth-weight infants and a higher likelihood of developmental problems, respiratory illness, and cerebral palsy. There are substantial risks to your health as well.

Women who carry twins, triplets, and quadruplets often experience potentially life-threatening complications during pregnancy. High blood pressure (preeclampsia) is three to five times more likely to occur in a

**A word to the wise:** | If you think that you might choose selective reduction if faced with a high-order multiple pregnancy, you might consider not telling friends and family members when you find out that you're carrying multiples. While the excitement is overwhelming and you want to share the news with everyone, if you do choose to reduce the pregnancy, you're exposing yourself to other people's opinions, criticism, and questions at a time when you are least able to deal with it. Given the personal nature of the decision to reduce a multiple pregnancy, you might want to keep it confidential, at least until you feel ready and able to address other people's opinions about your decision.

multiple gestation pregnancy than in a singleton (one baby) pregnancy and can be life-threatening to both mother and babies. The risk of premature labor, gestational diabetes, anemia, and cesarean sections are so high that most women carrying multiples are placed on strict bed rest, often in a hospital setting, for *months*.

Medical risks aside, there are also substantial emotional and financial risks connected with multiple births. Long-term hospitalization is often required for both mother and babies and isn't always completely covered by insurance. A premature infant can incur $100,000 in medical costs in just a few weeks. And the cost of caring for and raising multiples is overwhelming (and these costs come after expensive fertility treatments). Factor in the emotional strain of worrying about your pregnancy, not being able to live a normal life due to severe lifestyle restrictions, and the additional fatigue and higher hormone levels presented by a multiple pregnancy, and chances are good that the ordeal will leave you exhausted and strung out.

If you or your surrogate wind up with a multiple pregnancy of triplets or greater, your RE will probably ask you if you want to selectively reduce the pregnancy. With selective reduction, a highly trained physician terminates one or more of the pregnancies in order to increase the odds that the remaining pregnancies survive and thrive. It also reduces your risk of complications. After enduring years of heartbreaking infertility and profoundly challenging treatment, the last thing you want to do is have to think about, let alone undertake, a procedure designed to end a life. Though often rational, the decision to reduce a multiple pregnancy is heartbreaking and may haunt you for years to come. If you're faced with this decision, I encourage you to seek counseling from a therapist who specializes in these issues, and with a high-risk obstetrician or perinatologist (these guys specialize in dealing with multiple pregnancies and other complicated pregnancies) to fully understand what you're facing. This is a profoundly personal decision that should only be made after you've gathered a lot of information.

There are ways to reduce your risk of conceiving multiples. First, have a frank conversation with your RE about adequately controlling the stimulation phase of an IUI. For IVF patients, discuss with your RE how many embryos she believes can safely be transferred to your uterus without incurring a substantial risk of multiples. If you're young, discuss making blastocyst transfer (see chapter 12) a goal of the cycle.

You might also consider freezing embryos you don't need to use right away. Many couples choose to cryopreserve embryos to use on subsequent attempts at pregnancy. This gives you the option of creating siblings if your initial cycle—the cycle in which the frozen embies were created—results in a live birth. Most clinics have frozen embryo programs, although some are more successful than others.

There may come a day when your family is complete and you have frozen embryos you will not want to use. Your clinic will likely have you sign a consent form at the beginning of your IVF cycle that permits them to destroy the embryos at a certain point in time (usually around your fiftieth birthday) or donate them for research. But you do need to think about whether embryo adoption would be a better option for you.

Ovarian hyperstimulation syndrome (OHSS) is another serious risk of infertility treatment that cannot be overlooked. Most IVF patients don't experience it, but it's a real and potentially life-threatening complication. OHSS occurs when your body produces too many follicles (eggs) and your estrogen level gets dangerously high. The follicles secrete fluid (this is normal) after egg retrieval; in women with OHSS, so much fluid is secreted that the body cannot absorb it all. The abdominal cavity becomes extremely distended (it's filled with this fluid), sometimes making it difficult to urinate and breathe. You can go into renal (kidney) failure and/or need lifesaving emergency surgery to remove the fluid. Your clinic *should* give you a list of symptoms to watch out for after egg retrieval.

Women who are young, have PCOS, or aren't managed properly during their stims phase (see chapters 11 and 12) are at greater risk for developing OHSS. I had a cycle canceled as a precaution because my E2 level was so high that Dr. Chung was concerned about the risk that I would dangerously hyperstimulate after retrieval. Some less reputable clinics are very aggressive with stimulating patients and have higher-than-average rates of patients experiencing OHSS. Make sure the clinic you choose properly manages patients to avoid OHSS and watches carefully for OHSS symptoms!

When deciding on a course of treatment, don't overlook your emotional commitment and resources, your age, economic position, and the strength of your marriage. Make a game plan. Create a reproductive treatment map with the help of your RE. Analyze how much time, money, and energy you want to devote to this and figure out which option best fits with your resources. For each stop on your map, list alternatives.

I decided to start methodically. My plan was three cycles of IUI. If that didn't work, we'd move on to IVF. I got pregnant repeatedly and learned I couldn't stay pregnant. I didn't know what to do next. Whatever your situation, have a contingency plan. I was emotionally and physically exhausted and way too depressed to think about how to approach family building once I realized that medical treatment couldn't help me anymore. I took some time and reviewed my options, and with a surprising amount of relief and joy, I moved on to adoption. A contingency plan that included adoption would've been helpful, but at the time I didn't know to make one.

Do your research and take time to think and visualize what your life might be like with each treatment option (how would your life be if you got pregnant with triplets?). Figure out what is right for you and your partner, make your plan, and when you're ready (and have your care package all set to go), pick up that needle, adoption profile, or round-the-world cruise brochure and run (do not walk) toward your future!

# 8

## Telling Friends and Family

WELCOME TO LAND-MINE CITY!

It is amazing how many people decide not to tell anyone, *ever*, that they're undergoing infertility treatment. I understand why you want to keep this crisis in your marriage—heck, in your life—private and why you'd want to shut everyone out. You need time to absorb, adjust, and accept what is happening to you without people scrutinizing your every reaction and telling you what to do. But there comes a point when you will need support from other people. Support is extraordinarily important when you're struggling with infertility. Trust me; you won't be able to cope with this without help and support from friends and family.

Unfortunately, the decision to keep your infertility a secret usually backfires. First, your secrecy inevitably leads to feelings of shame and guilt. There's nothing wrong with being infertile. By keeping your infertility a secret, you cut yourself off from the love and support you need. Why feel more isolated than you already do? Worse, if you keep it all a secret, people will make unfair judgments about what you're doing and have expectations that you cannot meet or fulfill.

Many mothers have looked at their childless daughters and sons-in-law and presumed they were choosing to wait to have babies. This presumption usually leads to insensitive and intrusive comments and (of course) pressure. Mothers make comments about your ticking biological clock while you bite your tongue, dying to point out that not everyone can make a baby when they want to. Mothers-in-law jabber away about their younger son's beautiful new baby and how much she wishes for another grandbaby. She offhandedly observes that your brother-in-law is "way ahead of you" and that you really ought to think about trying to catch up (as if family building were some kind of race or competition). And don't you love the unspoken reminder that while your hubby may be the oldest, he was not the first to bless your in-laws with grandchildren? What is with this competition thing anyway?

Eventually, after months (or years) of coping with insensitive people, the resentment builds to volcanic proportion. You become a walking time bomb of rage and fury. You're dealing with the demands of infertility treatment, hopped up on hormones, and coping with constant barbs from family and friends who're in the dark about what's going on and so don't know any better. The resentment and frustration level mushrooms. One wrong comment from your sister-in-law and *boom!* You blow sky-high. *Not fun.*

Friends expect you to be happy for them when they tell you they're expecting number two (or, God forbid, number *three;* this one's really tough to cope with when you still don't even have number one). You will be expected to (joyfully) attend baby showers when the last thing you want to see is another pregnant belly, tiny little baby clothes, or women oohing and aahing over the soon-to-be mommy and her cute maternity outfit. You cannot and should not go through this charade. But because you're hiding your infertility, you've got no choice. Secrecy means you have to attend or offend. Even worse, secrecy ensures that you're not going to get any slack for being a tad moody about having to be there in the first place!

My life got much easier when I started telling people what I was going through. Once family members knew what was going on, they realized we'd probably been trying when they got nosy the first, second, and third times. One or two relatives even apologized for being insensitive (imagine my *shock!*). Friends stopped expecting me to be at their baby showers and offered to take me out to lunch to cheer me up. What a refreshing change!

Infertility is a lot like a chronic illness. People need to know about it because they need to know that you're going to have good days and bad days, days where you're going to the doctor constantly and obsessed with test results, and days where there's nothing in your head except the overwhelming fear that you will never have a child. One unexpected benefit of sharing your experience is that you will meet more infertile couples than you ever dreamed existed. Once I started telling people what I was going through, two women at work told me that they conceived their babies through ART, and three close friends admitted that they, too, were having difficulties conceiving. Friends started introducing me to other women struggling with similar problems. Through this infertility networking (there's something you didn't think of!) I made many new friends. There will be other benefits, too, but these are the big ones. If you decide to share your experience, you will find that people do understand and care about you. The question is with whom do you share, and when and what do you tell them?

## Who to Tell and What to Say

This is where it gets tricky. I recommend making a list of the different types of people in your life (it can be a mental list, this isn't terribly hard) and break it into categories of who gets full disclosure and who gets more limited information.

With the exception of your best girlfriend, I don't recommend disclosing every detail of every treatment cycle or step in your journey to parenthood. There was a funny and *real* moment during the first season of the CBS television series *Judging Amy*. During a family dinner, Amy's sister-in-law recounts the details of her latest IVF cycle. Amy's mother (Tyne Daly's character) gets fed up and says something like, "Oh for God's sake, I know more about her ovaries than I do my own!" This happens in real life, too. You want your mother (or mother-in-law) to know enough so that she stops asking intrusive questions and excuses you from family dinners when you're not feeling well. But you don't want her to get tired of hearing about your treatment (you want her support) or involve her so much she calls you on the day of your pregnancy test to find out if you're pregnant (and you thought the phone call was the clinic with the results of your pregnancy test).

Similarly, you want your boss to know something is going on so you don't have to be in the office every morning when you've got blood work and ultrasounds. But you don't want him to know so much that your privacy is violated or you get different treatment at work. Let's face it: you don't want your boss to know you might be taking maternity leave soon.

Remember, this is *your* experience. Controlling who knows what (and when), will help protect your privacy and the intimacy of the experience. Make sure the first person who finds out you're pregnant (other than your clinic) is your partner, not your boss or mother-in-law.

When Charlie and I were figuring out who we were going to share our experience with, we divided people we knew into categories based on the degree of intimacy of our relationship with them. For example, we made a list that included: family, good friends, social friends, co-workers with whom we're friendly, our bosses and human resources people at our jobs, and finally coworkers and acquaintances we barely knew (and maybe didn't want to get to know). Then we broke that list down further and identified how many details we'd share within each group or category. For example, we decided to share details of treatment with casual friends, but only after the fact. It really helped me when I bumped into someone at the supermarket who was asking how "things" were going. I'd run down my mental checklist (social friend: they don't hear any current details) and I'd know how to respond: "We're great! We're going on vacation and thinking about doing an IVF cycle after that! How are you?"

So now you've figured out which people in your life you're going to share your experience with. You'll soon see that you've reduced your overall stress level and will start receiving emotional support from people. Life will be easier, but let's be realistic, this is a tough situation, and you're

**A word to the wise:** | Be very careful when talking with your boss or human resources department. Bosses—even those you adore—are surprisingly unsympathetic. If you've got a mentor, by all means share small parts of your experience, in confidence, but avoid sharing too much information. The bottom line is that your boss is not going to be pleased to learn that you're trying to have a baby. Maternity leave is bad enough, but the fact that you're going to need time off before you get pregnant or while you're pregnant isn't good news. Even the most liberal, open-minded companies start discriminating against female employees when issues surrounding work and family arise. My recommendation is this: tell your boss and human resources department that you're undergoing medical treatment for a chronic, non–life-threatening illness; you may need some time off from work but will be able to work from home. Tell them that you may need flexible hours for a little while, but you'll be able to stay later in the evenings (do your shots later in the evening or in a locked bathroom or office) or make up the hours on the weekend. You may need a few days off from the office after a surgical procedure, but you'll schedule around it and make sure to meet all deadlines, etc. *Keep it simple, and let your boss know you're flexible and committed.*

going to feel raw and sensitive a lot of the time, even after you've come out of the infertility closet (the hormones you're injecting yourself with are enough to make you certifiable). You've diffused the major land mines by sharing your infertility with people, but there are still more out there.

## How to Cope with Insensitive Comments

No matter how on top of the situation you are, there will still be insensitive, condescending, thoughtless, opinionated, and otherwise annoying comments to contend with. There is the well-meaning but utterly *condescending* suggestion: "Did you try Dr. so and so? He's really the best, you know. My friend who could not get pregnant for years got pregnant on her first try with him! You should really go to him if you want to get pregnant." Dr. so and so is either a total quack or is one of the doctors in your doctor's practice, but you can't tell her that without inviting another discussion (which you don't want) about why he's really a quack or why you're staying with your doctor.

From those *opinionated* folks who're all too ready to tell you the perfect way to solve your infertility crisis, you'll probably hear something like: "I think it's time you considered adoption." That was one of my favorites! Especially when someone said that to me two weeks after a miscarriage—most excellent timing. If you can respond without crying (miscarriage or no miscarriage), you're way ahead of the game.

And of course there are the *just plain thoughtless* comments. I once overheard my mother talking to several extended family members about my "ordeal" with IVF. She told them that Charlie and I had tried IVF "again and again and again and again, and it never worked, nothing ever happened." Imagine my stupefaction! Were we even living in the same universe? It was bad enough to hear her dishing about my infertility, but she wasn't accurately characterizing the facts (and if she's going to violate my confidence, she should at least get the story straight!). Yes we tried IVF "again and again and again," but I got pregnant "again and again and again." To say, "nothing ever happened," completely misrepresented my experience and invalidated the particular hell I was living through.

What do you do when you get an insensitive remark from someone who knows about your infertility? You may not explode every time, but you're still going to be pissed off and hurt. There are a couple of ways to cope: learn to match your mood and the personality you're dealing with and you'll have an effective and satisfying system for dealing with crappy comments.

For example, one strategy is to try to shut the person up (for good if possible). The best way to do this is to agree with the comment-maker. The egghead who tells you what doctor to go to doesn't expect you to agree; she wants to have the pleasure of showing you that she's right and knows everything! Say something like: "Gee *thanks* for the recommendation. I'm really happy with my doctor, but John and I will definitely look into this doctor you've mentioned." That shuts her up real fast. She never expected you to take her advice! It's simple and surprisingly effective.

Another effective approach that requires more energy is to tackle the comment head-on. This helps clear up misconceptions, education/awareness gaps, and reminds people that you've got feelings. (They forget you have them, isn't that just too weird?) But for this to work, you need to have a pretty solid relationship with the person with whom you're going to interact. Educating an office mate who makes an insensitive comment isn't worth the time or energy this strategy requires; educating your mother is worth it! I usually wait until I've regained my composure (always important) and then address the person directly but in a calm, nonjudgmental, nonconfrontational manner (even if I'm imagining myself stabbing them with needles filled with Lupron). I explain that what they said upset me, and I explain why as clearly and simply as I can. Then I tell them what I would've preferred they'd said or done.

After I overheard my mother talking about my struggle, when she and I were alone (and I had calmed down), I told her that I found her remark extremely insensitive and invalidating. First I explained that it was my experience to share with other people. If, however, she was going to talk about it with people, she needed to be accurate. Talking to her made me realize how little my mother knew about what I was feeling and that I hadn't done a very good job of letting her know what information was okay to share and with whom. My mother felt absolutely horrible and was grateful that I'd talked to her about it. We were able to clarify a lot about what my privacy boundaries were and how I was feeling about my miscarriages.

You'll probably find that most of the time, when you confront someone, they will—as my mother did—apologize profusely for whatever insensitive remark they made. Occasionally, however, you'll get a defensive response. Someone will try to blame *you* for being upset (telling you that you're *too sensitive* and need to *get over it.* Yeah right!). In these situations, *walk away!* Nothing you'll say will make this person think about it from your perspective. (I usually add a few extra needles of Lupron to my imaginary arsenal. I never said I wasn't human!)

## How to Cope with Social and Work Obligations

You'll also still have to deal with baby showers, postbirth hospital visits, and the occasional bris or christening. Try getting out of social events without telling the world what you're going through! Not easy, is it? What should you do when someone who doesn't know what you're going through invites you to a baby shower? Or what do you do when you've got an office retreat in the middle of your cycle? A little creativity can go a long way in situations like these! This is a time when you can avoid a whole lot of emotional discomfort with a teensy little white lie. Got an issue with lying? *Get over it!*

You're going through a crisis and need to protect yourself and your emotional well-being at all costs. Your priority is *you,* not obeying the Truth God. Honestly, you don't think the Truth God will forgive you? The Truth God doesn't want to go to the baby shower any more than you do!

For *baby showers* that you don't want to attend, my recommendation (and that of my other infertile friends) is to RSVP in the affirmative, pretend that you can't wait to go, buy an extra nice present (guilt), and then when the big day arrives, suddenly come down with a flu. You can't get sick too often, so you may need to work suddenly or go out of town for a romantic weekend (and by all means, do get out of town!).

You can also be honest about what's going on (how novel!). I think the only time you can truly be honest is with close friends who know how much trouble you're having. One friend called to see if I wanted to help plan a baby shower for a mutual friend. She said that she'd heard I'd just suffered another miscarriage and that both she and the soon-to-

**A word to the wise:** | The last thing you need to do is subject yourself to shopping for that baby shower present in an actual store filled with pregnant women and screaming newborns. Find out where the mother-to-be is registered and see if you can buy something off her registry over the phone or on the Internet. Otherwise pick a good baby product store on the Web (someplace she can return stuff in person) and buy something on-line. Spend the extra bucks to have it gift wrapped (guilt again), and then send it (with gift card) to the location where the shower is being thrown (this adds to the authenticity that you were intending to be there all along). The present is taken care of with minimal stress and anxiety, you get the present to the party, and then all you have to do is send that note of apology. Slick, isn't it?

be-mom didn't want me to feel any pressure to attend the shower. They wanted me to know that they understood how difficult my experience was, but they didn't want me to feel shut out or excluded, either. I was moved by her honesty. I decided to be just as honest and said that, as much as I wanted to be a part of the shower, I could still barely get dressed in the morning or get through the day without crying. There was no way I could handle a baby shower. My friends understood and accepted this. It was the first guilt-free experience I ever had declining a baby shower invitation.

Whether you use a creative little white lie or are honest about why you're declining a baby shower invitation, send an apology note with your present after the party. The same strategies can be used with family social functions.

*Work obligations* are a little trickier. I had a laparoscopy scheduled for Labor Day weekend. I told my boss weeks ahead of time that I needed a few extra days off after the holiday; Charlie and I were taking a mini-vacation (I only had three weeks of accrued vacation time coming to me). The Thursday before Labor Day my boss informed me that he needed me to cover a court conference for him on the day after Labor Day. I reminded him I was going to be out of town. He told me to change my plans. I said I couldn't, and made up an excuse that my flight was nonrefundable and didn't get in until late at night. He told me to rebook the flight, and the firm would pay for it. At this point I had to confess that I wasn't going out of town but was having surgery. He didn't believe me! After a lengthy argument, I handed him the paperwork from my preadmission testing to prove that I was scheduled for surgery the following day. That wasn't fun.

This is why you want your office to know beforehand that you're undergoing medical treatment. If something comes up like a retreat, a court appearance, a major meeting with a client, or inventory (any kind of critical event that you normally cannot miss), you can explain that you're going to be in the hospital for an outpatient procedure, for some tests, or will be recovering from surgery. The nature of the treatment that keeps you from the critical office function is none of their business as long as they were forewarned. Hopefully, you won't have to show your boss your preadmission testing forms!

Despite my coping strategies, there's really no easy way to escape all the insensitive, obnoxious, and heartless comments you'll receive. No matter who you tell, how much you tell, or how much they love you, at some point someone will do or say something that hurts. One of my oldest friends disappeared from my life when she found out that I'm infertile; that really hurt. I guess some people feel guilty when they have what you want or they just aren't really friend material. The people who really care about Charlie and me stuck by us throughout this experience. One day when Charlie couldn't get out of work, my best friend came with me and held my hand during a diagnostic test. That's what friendship is.

And being open about the fact that I'm infertile also means that I've heard amazing stories of hope and inspiration. While waiting on line in CVS one day, my mother became besotted with a three-year old girl. My mother told the child's mother that her daughter was adorable. This woman started talking about her experience with infertility and how when, after seven years of trying, she was about to give up, she conceived. My mother—jaw on the floor—told her that I was going through infertility treatment: (This time it was okay for her to share!) The woman told my mother to tell me never to give up. When you're looking for signs to keep going, this kind of chance meeting is invaluable.

Honesty may be the best way to navigate your way through Land Mine City. When you're not hiding anything, you feel strong and good! You protect yourself from situations that are painful, you've warned the boss so that you can take necessary time off, and you can deal with people who don't get it. Yeah, you're going to step on a few land mines, and that's gonna suck! But at least you've done something to defuse the blasts.

# 9

# Affording Infertility

## EVEN MILLIONAIRES THINK THIS PART HURTS

Infertility is expensive! You realize this pretty quickly, but it doesn't sink in until you've been going through treatment for a while. It's one thing to send bills to your insurance company—or pay them yourself—for initial testing and maybe an IUI or two. But when you start big-time expensive treatment like IVF, major surgery like a laparoscopy, or you're on your fourth IUI cycle, your head starts to spin.

Let's take a look at an average infertility workup and initial treatment to get an idea. (I'll use my experience because I know approximately how much everything cost.)

| | |
|---:|:---|
| **OB-GYN visit, annual exam:** | **$150.00** (80% covered by insurance = out of pocket $30.00) |
| *Subtotal* | $ 30.00 |
| **Ultrasound:** | **$100.00** (100% covered by in-network insurance) |
| *Subtotal* | $ 30.00 |
| **Laparoscopy:** | **$9,750.00** (72% covered = out of pocket $2,750.00) |
| *Subtotal* | $2,780.00 |
| **Consult with RE:** | **$350.00** (60% covered = out of pocket $140.00) |
| *Subtotal* | $2,920.00 |
| **Hysterosalpinogram:** | **$600.00** (100% covered by in-network insurance) |
| *Subtotal* | $2,920.00 |
| **HIV testing:** | **$115.00** (60% covered = out of pocket $46.00) |

| | |
|---|---|
| *Subtotal* | $2,966.00 |
| **Semen analysis:** | **$200.00** (100% covered by in-network insurance) |
| *Subtotal* | $2,966.00 |
| **Cycle day 3 blood work:** | **$180.00** (60% covered = out of pocket $72.00) |
| *Subtotal* | $3,038.00 |
| **Pretreatment blood work:** | **$3,571.25** (60% covered = out of pocket $1,428.50) |
| *Subtotal* | $4,466.50 |
| **IUI blood work monitoring:** | **$735.00** (60% covered = out of pocket $294.00) |
| *Subtotal* | $4,760.50 |
| **IUI ultrasound monitoring:** | **$1,200.00** (80% covered = out of pocket $240.00) |
| *Subtotal* | $5,000.50 |
| **IUI meds:** | **$1,500.00** (50% covered = out of pocket $750.00) |
| *Subtotal* | $5,750.50 |
| **IUI procedure:** | **$500.00** (80% covered = out of pocket $100.00) |
| *Subtotal* | $5,850.50 |
| **Pregnancy test:** | **$285.00** (60% covered = out of pocket $114.00) |
| *Subtotal* | $5,964.50 |

Yep, by the time I'd made it through all my infertility testing and had my first IUI, I had already wracked up nearly $6,000 in *out-of-pocket* charges! And I had three more IUIs, another laparoscopy, a hysteroscopy, five completed IVF cycles, and two D & C surgical procedures (just to name a few really high-ticket treatments) before I called it a day. I saved some money by finding an RE who accepted my insurance for major surgical expenses, but I still had to pay for my IVF cycles and meds and pregnancy tests and pregnancy ultrasounds. I added it up the other day and, including expenses paid by insurance, we were billed over $85,000 for all our infertility treatment. That's my kid's college education (almost)! And then I had adoption expenses!

So how do normal people afford this? If you earn five million dollars a year, six thousand dollars doesn't seem like much. But believe me, even the five-million-dollar-a-year couple balks at spending eighty-five thousand dollars to have a baby. The good news is that there are more options for managing these horrific costs than you may think.

## The Ins and Outs of Health Insurance

Almost every state in the U.S. has laws about how much of infertility treatment insurance carriers must cover. Massachusetts and a few other states mandate insurance coverage for IVF. New York provides mandated coverage only for IUIs and medication. New Jersey provides mandated coverage for three IVF cycles. In states that don't have a mandated insurance coverage, companies are free to impose their own restrictions on coverage. Some refuse to cover any infertility testing or treatment at all. Others provide coverage up to $5,000, $15,000, or sometimes even $25,000. Your first step should be to find out what mandates your state imposes on insurance carriers (check with your local chapter of RESOLVE or AIA) and then read your insurance policy *very carefully*.

If you are lucky enough to have insurance that covers IUI, IVF, and other assisted reproductive technologies, make sure you get the most out of the coverage you have. It's important to understand what type of coverage you have and how much you have. Try, too, not to make some common mistakes that can result in your squandering precious insurance dollars. There are also a few ways to help make sure your insurance claims are reimbursed in a timely fashion. The world of insurance can be hard to navigate, but a few simple measures can help you get the most out of your policy.

If you have a copy of your insurance policy, *read all of it*, including all riders and addendums. Don't stop after the section on infertility treatment (assuming you can even find one) because there are other separate provisions that may apply, too. Be sure to read all the provisions that pertain to *exclusions* and *limitations*. Generally, the policy says whether it covers ART, but there may also be provisions that limit coverage (usually the dollar amount of coverage). These provisions may not be on the same page of your policy—or even in the same section—but read them together so you fully grasp what's covered and what isn't.

Sometimes a policy covers IUI but not IVF, or pays for IVF but only if performed at certain designated facilities. Or you may find that no matter what type of treatment you use, you get only $10,000 of lifetime coverage (including the cost of medication). Some policies cover ART but don't mention this in the contract because the company doesn't want to advertise the fact that it covers infertility. If you don't find language in your policy that applies to infertility treatment, don't assume that your insurance carrier doesn't cover treatment.

As you review your policy, make a list of what it says, and on what paragraph and page. This will help you keep track of things if you have to refer back and forth between separate sections of the policy or if you have questions later on and need to find the paragraph quickly.

Next you need to check to see whether there are any provisions that pertain to precertification requirements. Many policies require you to get certified in order to receive treatment. Some policies require you to prove you've got a medically documented cause of infertility *and* further require you to prove that you've been trying to conceive for a certain period of time before they pay for treatment. Some policies require you to get recertified every three months (as if your infertility would suddenly go away!). Make sure you know about and comply with these requirements. Your doctor's office may have someone who can take care of this for you (make sure you remind them to call your insurance carrier if and when you need to get recertified). It sucks to blow a precert deadline and then have to pay for a cycle out of pocket!

If you have any questions about what the language in your policy means (most insurance policies are not written in user-friendly English), you might want to ask someone to help. I recommend that even if you think you understand your policy, talk it through with an expert. So, who do you ask? Many people aren't comfortable asking their employer for clarification of IVF coverage. And it's possible your employer won't have the most up-to-date information about its coverage. As shocking as this sounds, insurance plans are subject to change without notice, and sometimes the carrier doesn't notify participants of changes to the policy. I made the mistake of relying on someone at my husband's company for information on how much infertility coverage we had. It turned out she was reading from an older version of the policy and didn't know that the coverage amount had been *reduced* by $10,000. It wasn't until I contacted the insurance carrier directly that I learned of the change. I was out of pocket a whole lot o' money. So you're probably better off contacting the insurance carrier directly, or someone who represents the insurance carrier (for example, you can call your employer's insurance broker) to make sure you understand your policy.

If you talk to the carrier directly, you can go over individual procedures (using the insurance billing, or CPT codes) and find out how much your insurance reimburses. This will help you get a sense of how much money might come out of your pocket (some carriers will require you to submit a list of CPT codes in writing before they will tell you what they will cover). Don't forget to take notes on your conversation (including the name of the person you spoke to, date, and time of the call) and get as many details as possible about the scope of your coverage. (Later in the chapter I give you a checklist that includes some things you might want to ask your insurance carrier.)

Now that you're familiar with the scope and requirements of your insurance coverage, you're ready to enter the world of HICF (pronounced *Hicfa*, if you want to sound in the know), or health insurance claim forms. These are the forms that you or your doctor submit to your insurance carrier for reimbursement. They specify the date and type of service, the cost of the service, and whether the service has been paid for (so you get reimbursed) or whether there is a balance (meaning the doctor has not yet been paid). Make sure you file these forms *as soon as possible* after you've paid for treatment so that you get reimbursed as quickly as possible. If your doctor is seeking reimbursement from your insurance, it's less important to you that the form gets filed quickly (you're not the one waiting for money). But you still want to stay on top of when the HICF gets filed, because you need to know how much of the available coverage you've spent.

Because most REs don't accept insurance, I'm going to assume that you're the one (not your RE) who's getting reimbursed by your insurance company. I'm also going to assume that you've got to pay for your treatment up front (before treatment begins), so you're concerned about making sure you get your insurance reimbursement check quickly.

You'll need your HICF to get to your insurance carrier. Some clinics forward your completed HICF to you directly; others will send the HICF to your insurance company. Either way, it's important to find out *when* the HICF is sent. Your RE may mail the HICF after each procedure is completed, or the office may wait until your entire cycle is finished and then mail out the HICF (this could be six weeks after you paid for the cycle). If you are tight on cash, you might want to arrange to pick up completed HICFs at your RE's office throughout your cycle so that you can submit them yourself on a rolling basis (as each procedure gets completed, you send the HICF to your carrier). Once you've got your HICF, photocopy it for your records and mail it to your insurance company pronto! Don't forget to make note of the date you mailed it.

Keep track of the time that elapses after you submit your claim. If you haven't gotten a reimbursement check or response to a claim within a couple of months, call the carrier and make sure that it received your claim and is processing it. Don't hesitate to harass your carrier for reimbursement when it's slow to pay up. Insurance companies drag their feet on claims so they get to keep your money for one extra day. They will make up excuses and play tricks; don't let them!

Also, don't accept your insurance company's denial of a claim. A little-known secret of the insurance industry is that carriers routinely deny valid claims because most people don't fight about it. Each time someone chooses not to fight, the insurance company gets to keep a little more money! If your insurer denies a claim, fight with them; the odds are that you'll win, especially if you can point to the language in your insurance contract that specifies your infertility coverage. I'm still fighting with one insurance carrier. I won't give up; I've filed three appeals so far on the claim at issue (three appeals are required before I can seek redress in the court system), and one of these days the carrier is going to realize it's cheaper to pay my claim than go to court over it (which I'm more than happy to do). I've won once, and I'll win again. Perseverance is the name of the insurance game.

Keep track of the procedures billed on each HICF submitted to your insurance carrier and how much each procedure cost. Stay on top of what the insurance company is paying and what it is ignoring or disallowing. Make sure you get paid for every procedure listed on your HICF and that you get an acceptable explanation as to why any claim is disallowed.

Also, make sure that you are being reimbursed at the proper rate. If, for example, your RE is not part of your insurance network, your insurance policy sets a rate at which it will reimburse you for out-of-network services. Generally, a carrier pays 50 percent, 70 percent, or even 80 percent of the usual and customary rate (UCR). UCRs vary by region, so ask your carrier whether you're being reimbursed at the national rate (which sucks if you're living someplace where medical expenses are higher than the national average) or within a certain geographic distance from your RE (this is much more fair if you live somewhere like New York City where medical care is exorbitantly expensive, but it costs your employer much more money). The amount you spend out of network is usually capped at a certain amount (for example $1,000); this is called your out-of-pocket deductible.

Once you reach your out-of-pocket deductible, your insurance company is supposed to pay you 100 percent of the UCR for each claim. Let's look at a hypothetical situation to see how this works in the real world (before your eyes glass over). Your out-of-network RE charges you $200 for a procedure. Your contract provides that you're entitled to be reimbursed at 80 percent of the UCR for this procedure. The UCR for this procedure is $100 (you've just lost $100). So you're entitled to $80 in reimbursement on your $200 charge (80 percent of $100 = $80). This $80 then gets applied toward your out-of-pocket deductible (we'll say your deductible is $500). Spend another $420 unreimbursed dollars with your RE, and you'll be entitled to the full $100 (the UCR) for this or another procedure.

Your insurance carrier will tell you how much of every claim is applied to your deductible in the explanation of benefits (EOB) it sends.

Do not depend on your insurance carrier to calculate your deductible. Insurance companies can, and do, make mistakes. Keep track of how much you think you have spent toward the deductible, and don't hesitate to challenge your insurance company if you think its total is incorrect. Once you meet your deductible, make sure you are paid at 100 percent of the UCR for each service. Again, familiarity with the terms of your policy helps ensure that you get the most out of your insurance.

Look for claims applied more than once toward your lifetime maximum. Keeping a list of the date, cost, and nature of the procedure helps ensure that your insurance company or RE's office doesn't accidentally bill you twice for the same service.

Finally, be alert to the total amount of money you have under your policy and how much of it you have spent. Don't ignore where you are in your ART spending. You can wind up out of pocket for the cost of an entire IVF cycle if you haven't stayed on top of your claims status; if you realized you were maxing out on coverage earlier, you could've found other ways of financing your treatment.

## Insurance Checklist

Here are some questions to get answers to and some tips on filing claims:

- What is your lifetime maximum of infertility coverage? Is it $0, $5,000, $10,000, $25,000, or an unlimited amount?

- What are the limitations on coverage? What's covered, what isn't, what needs to be certified, if anything?

- What is your out-of-pocket deductible?

- At what rate will your insurance carrier be reimbursing you? Is it 50 percent, 70 percent, or 80 percent of the UCR?

- Is your doctor's office or clinic an authorized provider in your insurance network?

- Make a list of procedures and dates of service and keep track of what is being submitted to your carrier and when it's being submitted.

- Periodically (I recommend once every two weeks) check to see what claims are outstanding and call your insurance company if more than six weeks have gone by without receiving notice of the status of the claim.

- Check your own records and that of your insurance company (this may require a phone call) to see how much of your lifetime maximum (if you have one) has been spent.

- Check to make sure how much has been applied toward your out-of-pocket deductible.

- Check to make sure you are being reimbursed at the appropriate rate (70 percent, 80 percent, or 100 percent).

## Shared-Risk or Money-Back-Guarantee Programs

In response to the numerous patients who don't have insurance coverage, many clinics now offer shared-risk or money-back-guarantee programs (they're the same thing). Don't think these doctors are altruistic saints helping you afford to have a baby. These programs bring them more patients, and they often make a greater profit on a shared-risk arrangement than traditional fee-for-service programs.

Shared-risk and money-back-guarantee programs work in two ways. The first type of arrangement you enter into with your clinic. You pay a large sum of money up front (a multiple of the cost of a single IVF cycle—$20,000 if your RE normally charges $8,000 for each IVF cycle) and, in return, the clinic guarantees that if you fail to get pregnant within three or four IVF cycles, they will give you back all or part of your money. Alternatively, your clinic may contract with a service that provides the same type of arrangement. In this case you pay the service, which in turn pays your clinic for medical services provided to you. Both the network of Advanced Reproductive Care physicians (ARC) and IntegraMed offer shared-risk programs (if you're interested in finding a physician who participates in either ARC or IntegraMed, I've listed contact information for these companies in the Resources section). ARC and IntegraMed systems minimize certain conflicts of interests that can arise when your clinic or RE shares risk. I'll discuss conflicts later in this section.

Not every patient who wants to use a shared-risk program will be able to. The medical criteria used to determine which patients are eligible can be offensive. First, in order to qualify, you're going to have to pass certain medical tests. If after your medical workup (including CD3 blood work, HSG, and ultrasound, which you pay for on top of the cost of the shared-risk fee) your RE determines that you're very likely to get pregnant with IVF, you'll probably be accepted into the shared-risk program. These tests help your RE determine how much of a risk she's taking; if you pass these tests, your RE knows that she'll probably never have to pay you money back. These requirements are offensive because most people don't pass the tests and don't fall within the medical parameters necessary to participate in the program.

Usually, age is the biggest factor in determining whether you can participate in a shared-risk program. For example, a clinic will accept a woman less than thirty-five years of age with severe endometriosis and perhaps male-factor infertility, too. A thirty-seven-year-old woman with mild endometriosis and male-factor infertility might be excluded from participating in the shared-risk program. It depends on how well she does on her CD3 blood work; if she has good results (low FSH for example), she likely still makes good eggs and is at lower risk for IVF failure despite her age. A forty-year-old woman with no medical problems except that dreaded diagnosis, advanced maternal age, is excluded. These are very rigid criteria, and many couples will be excluded from participating due to the complexity of their infertility diagnoses. (I rather doubt that Charlie and I would ever qualify.)

In response to the backlash against extremely preclusive shared-risk programs, some clinics are becoming more open and flexible. Some programs stagger the cost to permit older women or those with more complex diagnoses to cycle. You pay more to participate if you're over thirty-five ($16,500 as opposed to $13,000 for women younger than thirty-four), but you still get back a large percentage of your costs if you fail to get pregnant. Many programs also now accept couples who need to utilize egg donation, surrogacy, ICSI, and even PGD. If you're interested in participating in a shared-risk program, get on the Internet and do some research. Find clinics that meet your criteria (if you're over thirty-five, you need to find a program that accepts women over thirty-five) and compare their IVF success rates. This is a service offered to you, the infertility consumer, so do the research to find a shared-risk program that meets *your* needs.

Despite the changes to make shared-risk more inclusive to patients with complicated diagnoses, the bottom line remains: couples accepted into shared-risk programs are more likely to achieve pregnancy quickly with IVF. Because couples are so rigorously screened and have such a high likelihood of success, those who are accepted into the program may be getting bilked out of a lot of money (while the clinic makes a handsome profit). Shared-risk programs work to your financial benefit when you don't get pregnant right away and to your REs benefit when you do.

Shared-risk programs may ask you to pay as much as $25,000 (not including medication or the cost of prescreening tests) up front, but for that price you're guaranteed three or four fresh IVF cycles, as many frozen cycles as you have frozen embryos, and usually the benefits of ICSI, assisted hatching, and maybe even PGD (depending on what assisted fertilization and embryo diagnostic testing you may need). If you still haven't gotten pregnant, depending on the clinic, you'll get 80 percent to 100 percent of the $25,000 back. If you get pregnant on your fourth fresh IVF cycle after also undergoing two frozen cycles, your cost per attempt may be less than $5,000. However, most couples who participate in these money-back-guarantee programs wind up paying closer to $10,000 or more per attempt; not much savings (if any) off the traditional fee-for-service system. And some might lose a good deal of money, paying $20,000 or more for one IVF cycle if they get pregnant on their first IVF attempt. Let's take a look at how this might work in the real world.

Couples A, B, and C join the shared-risk program at the same clinic and pay $20,000. For that fee they are guaranteed three fresh IVF cycles, all the frozen cycles for which they have frozen embryos, ICSI, and/or assisted hatching if they need it. The cost of a normal IVF cycle at this clinic is $8,000, ICSI is $1,500, and assisted hatching costs $2,500. A frozen embryo cycle costs $3,500. We'll assume (to make the math easier) that the cost of all medicines is included in all the prices I've listed (like that would ever really happen!).

Couple A takes three IVF attempts to get pregnant and uses one frozen cycle. They also use ICSI on every attempt and assisted hatching once. Here's how the cost/benefit breaks down for Couple A:

**Shared Risk:**
Couple A spent $20,000

**Fee-for-service:**

| | |
|---|---|
| Couple A would have spent $8,000 × 3 = | $24,000 |
| + ICSI $1,500 × 3 = | $ 4,500 |
| + assisted hatching = | $ 2,500 |
| | $31,000 |
| + frozen cycle = | $ 3,500 |
| **Total fee-for-service cost =** | **$34,500** |

Couple A saves $14,500 by doing shared-risk!

Couple B fails to get pregnant from their first fresh IVF cycle but conceives on their second attempt using the frozen embryos created during the first (fresh) cycle. They also use ICSI. Here's how the cost/benefit breaks down for Couple B and their clinic:

**Shared Risk:**
Couple B spent $20,000

**Fee-for-service:**
Couple B would have spent

| | |
|---|---|
| $8,000 = | $ 8,000 |
| + ICSI $1,500 = | $ 1,500 |
| + 2 frozen cycles = | $ 7,000 |
| **Total fee-for-service cost =** | **$16,500** |

Couple B lost $3,500 by doing shared-risk!

The clinic profited on Couple B by $3,500!

Couple C conceives on their first cycle without using ICSI or assisted hatching. Here's how the cost/benefit breaks down for Couple C and their clinic:

**Shared Risk:**
Couple C spent $20,000

**Fee-for-service:**
Couple C would have spent

| | |
|---|---|
| $8,000 = | $ 8,000 |
| **Total fee-for-service cost =** | **$ 8,000** |

Couple C lost $12,000 by doing shared-risk!

The clinic profited on Couple C by $12,000!

This is what your RE is hoping will happen and why you've been screened so carefully (to give your RE the best chance this will happen). You may want to consider using a traditional fee-for-service arrangement if you're accepted into a money-back program as it may be less expensive for you if you get pregnant quickly ($8,000 for a fee-for-service arrangement versus the $20,000 you spent on a shared-risk program).

There are some infuriating little-known facts about shared-risk programs. Look at the way each program defines success. At some clinics success is defined as a live birth. If you miscarry (even repeatedly) you're still eligible to continue in the shared-risk program without losing money. Other clinics define success as a clinical pregnancy. If you miscarry after achieving a clinical pregnancy, you've lost the $25,000 you paid. Additionally, you'll want to know whether there are restrictions on how many cycles you can do in a specified period of time and how long a break you must take in between cycles. Some programs may only permit you to cycle twice a year and may only give you two years in which to complete the program. Some women may not be able to utilize all the attempts to which they are entitled with these restrictions. Can you really be expected to complete four fresh IVF cycles and maybe one frozen cycle with the downtime you might be forced to take in between cycles (while waiting for a spot in the next series or while recovering from a miscarriage) in two years? I don't think so!

Some clinics are really aggressive with patients in their shared-risk program. In an effort to ensure higher pregnancy rates (so they don't have to pay you back) the clinic transfers a greater number of embryos. This puts you at high risk for a high-order multiple birth pregnancy. The advantage of systems like ARC and IntegraMed is that your RE or clinic gets paid regardless of your cycle's outcome, so she's less likely to take risks with your medical care. You're also protected from the risk that your RE or clinic will go out of business before you get your refund. IntegraMed is a publicly held company with a reserve fund, and ARC is reinsured through Lloyd's of London.

Many shared-risk programs let you opt out after a certain number of tries and get back a portion of the $25,000 based on the services already performed. This is a great option if you decide that you cannot continue with treatment. Interestingly, some women are grateful for not having an opt-out provision in their shared-risk agreement. I have repeatedly read comments that the lack of an opt-out provision was a blessing because it pushed couples to continue treatment beyond the point at which they believed they could endure emotionally. On the next attempt—after they would have otherwise given up—they conceived!

You need to read the fine print on your clinic's shared-risk program before making any decisions about whether it's right for you. You must analyze exactly what services are included, what's offered at an additional cost, the timing of cycles and duration of the program, the goals of your cycle, and what happens if you choose not to participate or get pregnant and miscarry. Once you have examined these issues, you can better determine whether this is something that might help mitigate your infertility expenses.

## Other Ways to Save Money or Pay for IVF

Some clinics don't offer shared-risk programs but do have package deals. If you participate repeatedly, attempts at IVF become progressively less expensive. For example, your first two cycles may be charged at 100 percent of the clinic's rate, but your third attempt is billed at 80 percent, and your fourth attempt is billed at 70 percent. Alternatively, you can pay a reduced price for a multiple cycle package (for example $20,000 up front for three cycles instead of $30,000). There's no refund if you fail to achieve a pregnancy, but if you're looking at three or four cycles before you have a good chance of success (something your RE can help you determine), a package like this might save you money in the long run.

If your clinic doesn't offer a deal like this, don't be shy. *Ask them* if you could negotiate such an arrangement. Sometimes the clinic will agree to comp you (it's free, as in complimentary) for services like ICSI or assisted hatching. This can save you a couple of thousand dollars. Sometimes you can negotiate a payment plan. Many clinics don't tell you they will do this, but when you ask them directly, you find out they will work with you to help you afford treatment.

Some clinics offer patients low-interest loans through local banks. If your clinic isn't one of them, at least one independent lending institution offers an affordable payment plan to couples undergoing infertility treatment. The Family Fee Plan offers low monthly payments with low fixed interest rates (rates as of this writing are as low as 10.99 percent) and repayment terms up to sixty months to couples who qualify (see the Resources section for contact information).

Another often-overlooked mechanism that can help save you money on treatment is the use of employer-sponsored flexible spending accounts. Many companies permit you to set aside a portion of your pretax income at the beginning of the year. You can use the money in this account to pay for the medical expenses you incur that year.

Most financial planners will shudder at the thought, but another way to finance treatment is to dip into your 401(k) or other retirement plans. Some 401(k) plans let you take personal loans for medical expenses without incurring a tax penalty. When it's time to pay the money back, you've got the advantage of knowing you're paying yourself back (not a bank or relative). People take loans from their 401(k) plans all the time to help finance their homes. If your plan permits you to take a personal loan, using this money for baby-making is just as important in terms of fulfilling your dreams as buying a house.

If you own your own home and you're not already up to your eyeballs in debt, think about taking a home equity loan. It's your equity, and you can use it for whatever you want. Which would you rather use the money for, a new kitchen or a baby (or two)? It's a no-brainer! You also can refinance your mortgage. Some people take second or even third mortgages to pay for infertility treatment.

People also take out multiple credit cards to finance treatment. If you do this, do yourself a favor and keep rolling that debt over to a card with a 0 percent introductory APR to save some interest while you're chipping away at the debt.

# How to Handle Other Infertility
# Financial Nightmares

Many couples have knock-down-drag-out fights about how to pay for infertility treatment. Infertility treatment is hard enough. Toss in financial strain, and you've got the makings for divorce (I'm not being facetious). This is one time that having a contingency plan can help. If you've got a clearly mapped out plan for your treatment, it will be a little easier to negotiate the cost. Knowing your limits will help you determine how much financial exposure you're looking at. And this makes it easier to figure out how to get the money you need.

## LOSS OF INSURANCE COVERAGE

After we ran through our savings, Charlie and I begged, borrowed, and practically stole money to be able to pay for treatment. We also learned to be flexible and creative. Twice we used federally mandated COBRA insurance coverage to maintain our existing policies. COBRA, which stands for the Consolidated Omnibus Budget Reconciliation Act (catchy title!) 29 U.S.C. §§1161-1169 (1989), lets you keep your insurance for up to eighteen months after you leave a job. You pay the insurance premiums yourself, but you have something like sixty days from your last day of employment in which to elect to use COBRA. This buys you some time when you're starting a new job to see if your new company's insurance covers infertility treatment.

When COBRA was no longer an option, I declared myself self-employed. After researching various bar association–sponsored insurance plans and plans offered through women's and writer's organizations (even if you have to join some kind of business association, this can be a great way of finding insurance), I found a new insurance policy that offered coverage for infertility and got a private policy that covered Charlie. It was expensive but offered us unlimited coverage for infertility testing and treatment.

One of my friends negotiated with her boss to allow her to participate in the insurance plan her company offered its executives (it offered coverage for IVF). She offered to pay the difference between the cost of the HMO (no infertility coverage) and the PPO (with infertility coverage) offered to executives. She promised not to tell anyone at the company she was doing this, and her boss allowed her to participate in the PPO.

When another of my friends hit the limit on her coverage under her health plan, she and her husband enrolled in his company's plan. It was more expensive, as her hubby's company made them pay the full cost of a family plan, but they got an additional $10,000 of coverage.

## PAYING FOR MEDICATION

Another friend had a policy that didn't cover medication. She enrolled in a free research study sponsored by a drug company; it paid for all her medication. Many clinics participate in studies sponsored by drug companies; this can be a great way to finance the cost of all or part of an IUI or IVF cycle. Similarly, larger research-based infertility centers sometimes accept patients into research studies for new treatments or techniques. If you qualify and don't mind being a guinea pig, these can be great ways to finance treatment. Check with your RE or clinic to see what studies are scheduled (or ongoing) and whether you can participate.

Donated drugs offer another way to help obtain medication. Oftentimes patients will donate unused, unopened meds to their RE's office or clinic when they achieve a pregnancy. Although this is illegal in some states, sometimes IVF nurses make medication available to patients who need it. If your insurance company won't cover the costs of your meds or only covers half of the amount you will need for your cycle, let the nursing staff know. They may be able to provide donated meds.

Do not under any circumstances ever purchase medication from an *individual* over the *Internet*. It is okay to purchase meds through an online pharmacy, but it's never advisable to buy medications from another patient. There is no way to know whether the medication was stored properly, has passed its expiration date, or has been opened and used. And there is no recourse in the event that you purchase inactive, adulterated, or expired meds from a stranger. Putting aside these risks, it's *illegal* for an individual to buy and sell prescription medications.

By all means use an on-line pharmacy or one located across the country from you; some of the best prices for infertility meds can be found on-line or in distant states. I've listed a few pharmacies in the Resources section that my friends and I've used. Your RE will have to fax a prescription to them, but it may be cheaper to do this than go somewhere local to obtain your meds. Pharmacies specializing in infertility (like Apthorp Pharmacy in New York City, which fills infertility drug prescriptions all over the United States; see the Resources section), offer better prices than your local chain pharmacy. And check with your insurance carrier to find out if it has a mail-order service that you can use to obtain fertility meds at a discounted rate (or perhaps even completely covered by insurance).

Paying for treatment and drugs isn't the only problem you might encounter. How on earth are you supposed to juggle the demands of your job with intensive, time-consuming treatment?

### TIME OFF FROM WORK

If you're having trouble managing the stress and time demands of infertility treatment with your work schedule (join the club), speak to your employer about taking a leave of absence and going on disability. Most employers will accommodate you. But if your boss gives you a hard time, there is a legal basis for the argument that infertility is a medical disability (I've given you a link that describes these cases to you in the Resources section). You will be able to collect your salary for a period of time and have some time off from work in which to pursue treatment singlemindedly. You can also use accrued vacation and personal days or ask to take unpaid leave.

If you think you'll need to quit altogether—as I did—see if there's a way to work part time somewhere low stress or do contract or temporary work to help offset the lost income. Several of my friends got part time jobs in department stores or places like Blockbuster and Bloomingdale's. They got discounts when they shopped (always a bonus), had something low-stress to do with their days, and made a little money to help with the bills. Alternatively, you could start a home-based business as I did.

Almost everyone goes into debt or spends their nest egg to finance treatment. You're not the only one spending money on family building that you've carefully saved and invested for other things. Most of us get the family we dream of but suffer a long-term financial crunch as a result. It sucks. Even millionaires think it sucks. Be creative. Think outside the financial box, and you'll come up with a way to pay for this.

# 10

# Becoming Your Own Advocate

YOU GO, GIRL!

Infertility treatment is horribly overwhelming. Your first urge may be to crawl under the covers and stay there until someone tells you that you're pregnant or otherwise delivers a baby to your doorstep. As tempting as this may be, you *cannot* do this! If you want to survive your infertility without getting smashed flatter than a pancake by a steam roller with your clinic's name on it (although some women might say that starting a pregnancy flatter than a pancake is a good thing), you're going to have to turn into an infertility activist, an advocate, a bulldog, a lioness, a dragon tamer—pick your image!

Infertility clinics are busy places where patients get lost in the shuffle. Overwhelmed nurses forget to make phone calls with evening medication dosage instructions and write wrong things on medical charts. Mistakes like these can result in pure mayhem. Usually, some nurse or doctor figures out that a mistake was made, but unless you're on top of the situation, errors probably will be discovered too late, and you'll be the one who suffers. Your cycle will be blown to Mars, and you can forget making a baby for a few months.

Seriously, I have friends who are incredibly intelligent, gutsy women, but when it comes to infertility, they turn into complete wusses. They don't want to deal with any of it. As a result, they assumed it was normal when they didn't get their evening phone calls with dosage instructions (no, you should get a phone call *every single night* of your cycle except maybe the night before retrieval or insemination! We'll talk about this in greater detail in chapters 11 and 12) and gave themselves the wrong dosage of meds, totally screwing up their cycle. Or they ignored something that didn't make sense and found out days later that they had been giving themselves the wrong combination or amount of medicine and had their cycle canceled. I'm a trained litigator, and I freaked out when I had to confront the doctors and nurses in my clinic (Charlie kept reminding me these people aren't God, but that didn't seem to diminish the intimidation factor one bit).

When I was doing my frozen *embryo* cycle, the nurse who went over the instructions for the cycle wrote in my chart that I was doing a frozen *blastocyst* transfer. The difference is rather significant. The transfer of a thawed blastocyst occurs on average two days later than for a frozen embryo, so the timing of medications to prepare you for transfer is different. I had the correct instructions in the handout she'd given me, but when I got closer to transfer, one night I got instructions different than those specified on my written instructions. It took five phone calls before the head nurse (who had to be called at home) figured out that I was doing a frozen embryo cycle and not a frozen blastocyst cycle, and I should follow the written instructions.

When it was all sorted out, I had a good cry with Charlie. It had been really tough to challenge these people. Yelling at another lawyer was one thing, but standing up to a *doctor* was something entirely different. This man had the power to give me a baby. I didn't want to piss him off, and I didn't want to create an incident, but I didn't want to lose out on the cycle, either.

*You have to stand up for yourself, because no one else is going to.* Here are my suggestions for how to be your own advocate.

Get a complete copy of your medical records and know what's in them. After each cycle is completed, ask for a copy of the paperwork from the cycle (blood test results, stimulation sheet, embryo report, pregnancy test results, everything!). Know what's going on every step of the way, and know what the next step is supposed to be. If there's ever a question about whether you've had a test or treatment, you'll have the answer (and refer them to the paperwork that proves it). Knowing that you've already had the $1,500 in prescreening IVF blood work saves you a second go-round when you tell a nurse, "I don't know, I think so," and she says, "Well let's do it again, anyway, just to be sure." You'll save yourself $1,500 of your precious insurance dollars (and about a pint of blood) repeating the blood tests.

Get educated! Find out everything you can about your diagnosis. Ask your RE questions. Hit the Internet and the library. Call RESOLVE, AIA, and ASRM for their fact sheets on whichever reproductive disorders are applicable to you. Talk to other patients. Once you know what's going on with your body, you can take a more active role in your treatment and can discuss treatment options with your doctor.

Find out how your clinic works. Who schedules cycles, who makes sure all your paperwork is complete, who handles billing? Make sure you know who the people are that you need to interact with and when you need to interact with them. If your clinic has a waiting list for patients to start their IVF cycle, make sure you know who and when to call to get yourself on that list. If you (God forbid) find out your cycle was unsuccessful, get on the phone with the cycle coordinator and get your name on the list for the next available IVF cycle! You can always change the date to a later cycle if your doctor wants you to take a break between your IVF cycles. But if your RE gives you the go-ahead to cycle right away, and you've waited the three weeks it took to get in to see your RE to discuss whether you should do another cycle, that could mean you don't get on the wait list and have to wait three months to cycle in the next available IVF series.

Start thinking about this as a consumer business (which it is). Your doctor may be exceptionally skilled, but she's not God. You're paying her a ton of money to provide you a service. You deserve good medical care and good personal treatment. Accept nothing less. Are there any circumstances in which you would pay someone tens of thousands of dollars and permit them to make mistakes, do a sloppy job, or treat you like crap? There shouldn't be!

Stand up for yourself when you're not treated appropriately, but try not to make any enemies when you do it. It's important to be clear, communicate directly, and express yourself completely. However, things are going to get tough, and you're going to be hyped up on major mood-altering hormones. It will be very easy to take your rage and hostility out on the nurse standing in front of you. *Never, ever* vent in the direction of your IVF nurse or anyone on staff at your infertility clinic. If someone makes a legitimate mistake (as happened to me in my frozen cycle), take it up with your RE and let her handle it.

On my first IVF cycle, I was a little late for my morning blood work. No one had told me that blood work monitoring started and finished earlier for IVF patients than for IUI patients. The nurse taking my blood that morning really let me have it! She must have spent ten minutes telling me over and over and over again that I was *late,* and this *could not happen again,* yada yada yada! I understood the first time she said it. By the third or fourth time she was repeating herself, I was getting a little pissed off; and I'm not especially nice when I'm angry (I think it's a lawyer thing). As patiently and politely as I could, I told her over and over again that *I didn't know* that I was supposed to be there earlier and that it *would never happen again* (although of course it did)! By the end of the conversation, we were both glaring at each other and wanted to kill! We laugh now about how we got off on the wrong foot, but it was close. This nurse was not someone I wanted to have as an enemy at my clinic!

If you're not used to standing up for yourself, start with baby steps. If someone says something that bothers you or something happens that isn't acceptable to you, speak up. Tell your RE (or whomever else would be appropriate to complain to) that you're unhappy! It's that simple. You've taken your first baby step! You go, girl!

You will see results when you express yourself, but that wasn't why you did it. You stood up for yourself because you needed to let someone know that your needs had not been met. This is a huge step toward being that dragon tamer! The next time something happens that displeases you (hopefully there won't be a next time), baby step number two is to speak up and ask someone to fix the problem. Even if you don't get what you asked for, you told someone exactly what you expect from your caregivers in the future. Baby step number three might be asking for your money back. Hello, girlfriend! When did you become a dragon tamer extraordinaire?

You can be smashed flat as a pancake, fight flames like a dragon tamer, or find something somewhere in between. It's your choice how you will experience your infertility treatment. The only thing I can promise you is that you will feel better and stronger if you choose the dragon taming path. You might even get to your baby faster because you avoided unnecessary medical mishaps and, together with your caregivers, made smart decisions. You go, girl!

# 11

# Understanding Your Cycle

### INFERTILITY TREATMENT EXPLAINED FOR
### NON-ROCKET SCIENTISTS

Congratulations! You've made it through all the tests and, perhaps, surgeries to finally get to this long-awaited day: the day you have new hope of conceiving a baby (or two or three) with help from the best medical science has to offer. I know it's hard to face the fact that you aren't going to do this the old-fashioned way (I was pretty angry about this for awhile), but it's also exciting to have hope again. Let's face it, after months of failing to conceive on your own, you were starting to panic. Now you know what's going on with your infertility and have decided on a treatment plan. It's time to get back into a mode of excitement and optimism, because this process is physically demanding!

This chapter is devoted to demystifying all of the quirks in infertility treatment. Here comes the white lab coat again. Sorry, this *is* a technical chapter (*yawn*); but I figure when it comes to needles and your body, you might want some technical information! Let's start with the hard stuff, the drugs (and not the good kind, either).

## Medications

**What it is:** All infertility patients who undergo ART procedures take medication to stimulate the growth of eggs; it's called *follicle-stimulating hormone* (FSH). The term FSH gets used in a couple of different contexts in this book (you'll recall from earlier chapters that we've already talked about the FSH your body makes). To avoid confusion, I'm going to refer to FSH medications as "stims," because they *stimulate* the growth of eggs. (If you're interested, you can read in the Appendix about how FSH and other hormones make eggs grow.)

Keep in mind that—as far as medication is concerned—there are two important differences between IUI and IVF cycles. In an IUI cycle you take less stims than in an IVF cycle. During an IUI cycle, your doctor tries to help you achieve a healthy ovulation of only about two or three eggs, while in an IVF cycle she wants to induce an even greater ovulation (called controlled ovarian hyperstimulation), of as many as ten eggs (or more). Making more eggs usually involves more medication. In addition to stims, IVFers take two other medications. There is a lot at stake financially and emotionally during IVF; to make sure you get the best possible response from your cycle, your RE will completely shut down your reproductive system so she can control everything herself with the stims. This additional IVF medication stops your body from making *any* hormones (this is called suppression). Then, after your eggs are surgically removed, IVFers take injections of supplemental progesterone (and sometimes estrogen as well) to support any developing pregnancy (their bodies will not know to make any hormones as a result of being suppressed). IUI patients may also get progesterone support (it will be in either pill or suppository form), but there are many clinics that don't prescribe it at all.

**What's involved:** Most stims are injected subcutaneously (into skin, sub-Q) or intramuscularly (into muscle, IM. Sounds great, doesn't it?). Sub-Q injections are performed with little tiny baby needles and usually don't hurt too much (thank God!). IM injections are done with bigger needles (big enough to cause this IVF patient a moment of pure horror the first time she saw one) and are injected into deep muscle like your gluteus maximus (your butt). They tend to be a little painful (sometimes they *really* hurt). If you care how big the needle is and how painful the injection is, then take note of the distinction. You may want to talk to your doctor about using drugs that are injected sub-Q instead of IM. If needles don't bother you, knowing which size needle goes with which injection comes in handy when you're doing injections of multiple drugs; some will be IM and some will be sub-Q. One stim, Clomid, is taken in pill form.

A breakdown of more commonly used stims appears on page 188. There are medications that aren't listed (and new medications come on the market all the time), so don't worry if the medication you're prescribed isn't represented here.

Clomid is often given as a first-line treatment in infertility. Before you go high-tech with IUI (or super high-tech with IVF), your doctor may try a few cycles of Clomid. However, Clomid has certain drawbacks, which you need to be aware of. First, taking Clomid for more than three months without a break can impair cervical fluid (which can hinder the ability of the sperm to reach and fertilize your egg in a natural conception) and cause the uterine lining to thin, which can reduce the chances of achieving a healthy implantation of the embryo. Because of these side effects, prolonged use of Clomid results in reduced pregnancy rates, which explains why the vast majority of Clomid pregnancies occur during the first three cycles of the drug's use.

Second, because Clomid is taken orally and acts directly on the brain, your doctor cannot control your response to it. One doctor I spoke to likened Clomid's effect on the brain to the detonation of a bomb; once it goes off, there's no going back and no way to shut it off (injectable stims can be controlled by reducing or increasing your daily dosage). Also, Clomid often doesn't work well for women over forty. Lastly, and perhaps most frightening if it happens to you, Clomid can cause temporary

| Medication | Purpose | Pill | Patch | Suppository | Nasal Spray | Sub-Q Injection | IM Injection |
|---|---|---|---|---|---|---|---|
| Antagon | Suppression | | | | | yes | |
| Climara | Hormone (estrogen support) | | yes | | | | |
| Clomid | Stim | yes | | | | | |
| Fertinex | Stim | | | | | yes | yes |
| Follistim | Stim | | | | | yes | |
| Gonal-F | Stim | | | | | yes | |
| HCG (human chorionic gonadotropin) | Final maturation of follicle for ovulation or retrieval | | | | | yes | yes |
| Humegon | Stim | | | | | yes | yes |
| Lupron | Suppression | | | | | yes | |
| Metrodin | Stim | | | | | yes | yes |
| Pergonal | Stim | | | | | | yes |
| Progesterone | Hormone support | yes | | yes | | | |
| Progesterone in oil | Post–embryo transfer hormone support | | | | | | yes |
| Repronex | Stim | | | | | yes | yes |
| Serophene | Stim | yes | | | | | |
| Synarel | Suppression | | | | yes | | |

blurred or double vision. If this happens to you, contact your doctor immediately! It will go away, but your doctor needs to know what's going on.

Because of the side effects and because your doctor can't regulate your response to Clomid, many physicians prefer to use injectable medications during IUI cycles (Clomid is not used in IVF cycles). Clomid can be used in combination with injectable stims like Gonal-F and Follistim. Most clinics, however, prefer to only use a low dose of an injectable stim like Gonal-F during an IUI cycle.

If you're taking Clomid to assist a natural cycle or for an IUI, you'll begin taking it on cycle day (CD) 2 or CD3 and continue for three, five, or seven days. It is taken in varying doses (50 mg, 100 mg, 150 mg) depending on how well you're expected to or have already responded to the medication.

Injectable stims are used more frequently with IUI (and exclusively with IVF) because doctors can better control your response to the drug (by varying doses and combinations of drugs). Also, because these stims have different compositions and act on the body in different ways, they can be effectively used to treat a variety of different problems.

Two important hormones are involved in the production of healthy eggs: FSH (follicle-stimulating hormone) and LH (luteinizing hormone). Both exist naturally in your body (some of the blood tests you've been having measure the amounts of these hormones in your body at various points in your menstrual cycle) and help you make eggs. Because your body responds differently to FSH and LH, some of the injectable stims contain both FSH and LH (for example, Pergonal contains both), while others contain only FSH (like Follistim and Gonal-F) or LH (Repronex). A mix of FSH and LH better mimics natural ovarian stimulation for some women and can help improve egg and embryo quality. Some of the stims are *purified* forms of FSH taken from the urine of menopausal women (nuns, I think). In contrast, there's *recombinant* FSH, which is created from bacteria using genetic engineering. For some women the recombinant form may be more bioactive (available to your body, easier to metabolize) than the purified form.

Your doctor will determine which stim or combination of stims will most benefit you. If you do more than one cycle, she might even switch to a different combination of FSH and LH stims the second (or third, or fourth) time around. I have taken Clomid, Follistim, Gonal-F, and Re- pronex. I never noticed a difference between the drugs or in my response to them (except I hated the Clomid and wasn't too fond of injecting Follistim; we'll talk about why later); but then again, white lab coat not- withstanding, I'm not a doctor.

Whether you're doing IUI or IVF, your dosage of stims will be based on your body mass index, medical condition (endometriosis, premature ovarian failure, PCOS, etc.), hormone levels on CD2 or CD3 of a natural cycle, previous response (if any) to stims, and the kind of response your doctor wants from your ovaries. Please *do not* read anything into the dosage of stims you're prescribed or compare it to what anyone else is prescribed. Everyone's dosage and protocol is different.

If you're doing IVF, you're also going to be taking meds to suppress your menstrual cycle. (More drugs, aren't you *so* happy to hear this?) Three of the drugs most commonly used to suppress ovulation are Lupron (an injectable), Synarel (a nasal spray), and Antagon (an injectable).

You inject stims once or twice a day, usually in the evening (some clinics may ask you to do one injection in the morning and another at night). If you're doing IUI, you can expect to have one injection a day, probably in the evening. If you're doing IVF, you may have as few as one injection a day or as many as four (horrible, I know). Before insemination or egg retrieval, you'll get an injection of HCG (human chorionic go- nadotropin) to ensure the timing of ovulation in relation to insemination, or final maturation of the egg in relation to retrieval. HCG causes the eggs to finish ripening and causes you to ovulate approximately thirty-six hours after the injection of the medication. The dosage is based on your E2 (estradiol/estrogen) level the morning before the HCG shot. This injection is usually done IM, but some clinics let you do it sub-Q. It has to do with absorption of the HCG; some clinics feel it's better absorbed into muscle rather than skin.

After your IUI or egg retrieval procedure, you may get progesterone and/or estrogen support. In an IUI cycle your RE may want to ensure that your body has sufficient quantities of progesterone to support a pregnancy (this may be overkill, but why take a chance, right?), so she may prescribe progesterone (pills or suppositories) to help you along. During an IVF cycle, your body doesn't make progesterone, so your RE *must* prescribe hormonal support to help an early pregnancy develop. Some REs prescribe both estrogen and progesterone for IVF patients; others use just progesterone. Some doctors feel progesterone suppositories are sufficient, while others will make you take injections of progesterone in oil (known among IVF patients as PIO, and it isn't fun stuff to inject).

## Protocols (IVF Only)

**What it is:** Every clinic and RE has a predetermined combination of drugs they use to stimulate egg production. The dosage of drugs varies for each patient. Basically there are two IVF protocols, the long "down-regulation" protocol and the "boost" or "flare" protocol.

**What's involved:** If your RE prescribes the *down-regulation protocol*, you'll begin taking medication to suppress your menstrual cycle (Lupron or Synarel) in the menstrual cycle preceding your IVF cycle. About a week after you ovulate, you'll begin injecting Lupron or sniffing your Synarel. For ease of reference, I am just going to talk about Lupron, but the response should be the same with either drug.

Depending on your clinic's preference, you'll get a dose of Lupron, injected sub-Q (the skin of your lower abdomen is easiest) every day. About seven to twelve days after you begin taking Lupron, you'll get what's know as a Lupron bleed, which is basically a *very heavy* period. I heard of one woman who had to line her car seat with garbage bags to prevent her from staining the seat on her drive home from work. Hopefully, your Lupron bleed won't be this bad (mine never were this bad, but they can be pretty gross).

Lupron scares a lot of people. It has a nasty, nasty reputation for vicious side effects. Taking Lupron can be tough, but the drug's reputation is a little unwarranted. I have taken Lupron seven times, and some cycles were very bad, and others were fine. Side effects range from bloating to severe bloating (most women can expect to gain about five pounds; some will gain more and others less), headaches and/or migraines (I believe this is due to dropping E2 levels), rashes, insomnia, difficulty concentrating and speaking coherently (again I think this is due to dropping E2 levels; I call this side effect "Lupwon bwain"), and mood swings. But bloating and headaches are most common. Apparently, Synarel has fewer side effects, but it's used less frequently. I am told this is because some infertility centers feel it's less reliable in inducing the suppressed state (I have no idea if this is medically accurate; as far as I'm concerned, this is a subject for doctors and scientists to debate, and I think you're lucky if you get spared any injections).

In the *"boost"* or *"flare"* protocol you'll begin taking Lupron (or another drug, for example, Antagon) on CD2, the day before you begin taking stims. You will take a lower dose of Lupron (a microdose) and will only take it for a few days. You should have fewer side effects than women who take larger doses and for longer periods of time. Women with high baseline FSH on CD3 (remember that CD3 blood work?) or who've responded poorly to stims in the past will likely be placed on this protocol. Additionally, women who've had good response to the drugs but poor egg quality may be put on this protocol, as the lower dosage of Lupron may improve egg quality in some women.

There is one more protocol that involves taking birth control pills (BCPs) in the cycle prior to the IVF cycle. Women likely to hyperstimulate or produce great numbers of eggs are often placed on this protocol to obtain a little extra suppression. Your RE may prescribe BCPs to help synchronize your menstrual cycle with your clinic's series calendar (I talk about series calendars in chapter 12). On this protocol, BCPs are taken in the cycle before your IVF cycle and are usually (but not always) used in conjunction with a microdose of a drug like Lupron. BCP protocols are not as common as they used to be. There may be some risk of oversuppression and problems with E2 levels plateauing (when they should be rising) later in the cycle. If you've got concerns about taking BCPs, talk to your doctor.

Now that you understand what you're putting into your body and why, let's talk about doing an injection and how you'll feel afterward.

## Injections

**What it is:** This nasty job—necessary to make eggs—requires you to stick needles filled with high-powered hormones into various parts of your body.

**What's involved:** Where you administer your injections depends on which stim you're taking and what your RE prefers. For example, Pergonal is usually injected IM in your rear end. Repronex can be injected either IM or sub-Q. Follistim and Gonal-F are usually injected sub-Q. The table on page 194 discusses where and how to do your shots.

Most women aren't able to do IM injections by themselves and need a husband, partner, or nurse (you'll probably have to pay the nurse) to help. Sometimes women have to do IM injections themselves due to travel plans (flying home solo from a clinic that's far away from home, husband's business trip, etc.) or trust issues. (Won't let hubby near you with a needle that big? I can relate!) I strongly encourage you to arrange to have someone else do this injection whenever possible; in a pinch, though, it's good to remember that women can do this shot themselves (this *really* blows my mind!).

Thicker IM injection medications like progesterone in oil, which is used after embryo transfer, are more difficult to inject. It is important to warm the vial of oil (stick it in your armpit for about ten or fifteen minutes before preparing the syringe), as warmer oil is easier to inject into tough muscle tissue. You will need to ice your derriere for this injection (while you might discover some of the other medications don't

## IM (intramuscular) Injection

### WHERE YOU DO IT

All IM injections should be done in your tush, in the upper and outer quadrant of your gluteus maximus. To find this spot, you can take a pen and divide your butt cheek in half (between your crack and your hip) and then cross that line horizontally from the top of your crack over to your hip. The upper right box created by that cross is where you'll do the injection.

### HOW TO DO IT

For IM injections you should use the non–needle-bearing hand to slightly stretch the skin between the index finger and thumb (sometimes this helps reduce the pain from the needle stick). Don't pretend to throw a dart; just pretend the needle is a pen and you're going to dot the period at the end of a sentence with a flourish! Quick, definitive, and to the point (pardon the pun)! After getting the needle in, stabilize the syringe with your nondominant hand, and use your dominant hand to draw back slightly on the syringe's plunger to make sure you haven't hit a vein. If blood comes back into the syringe, you need to start over (with a fresh syringe). You don't want to draw back too much, just enough to see that there is no blood return. If there is no blood return, depress the plunger on the syringe to gradually release the medication. Once the medication has been injected, the needle should be pulled out straight, and slight pressure should be applied to the injection site.

### TIPS FOR DOING IT

IM injections are best done lying down, as this ensures your glute (butt) muscle is completely relaxed. If for some reason you're doing it standing up, make sure you stand on the leg that is *not* receiving the injection, relaxing your other leg (it should be bent at the knee slightly) and hip into the standing leg. If you're doing it yourself, get naked (you don't want the elastic on your underwear snapping up in the middle of the injection!) and sit in a chair that you can twist around in easily (so you can reach the outside of your butt). Whether lying, standing, or sitting, you should try icing the area for a few minutes before doing the injection (I recommend lying on a reusable ice pack), as it will reduce the pain from the needle stick (it's usually painless if you ice). A good needle-stabber (like Charlie became after some practice) can even do a painless injection without ice; it's all in the technique.

For tips on preparing the syringe and greater detail on performing an injection, please check out the Appendix.

## Sub-Q (subcutaneous) Injection

### WHERE TO DO IT

You can do Sub-Q injections into a pinch of skin on your lower abdomen on either side of your belly button and just below it, your upper thigh, or the fleshy part of your hip.

### HOW TO DO IT

You just kind of poke yourself, but *definitively*. The motion is quick and decisive. Grab or pinch a fold of skin and then quickly jab. Pull the needle out straight, and gently massage the area or apply pressure.

### TIPS FOR DOING IT

If you experience any pain from doing a sub-Q injection you can try icing the spot before you do the shot. Don't ice for too long, just enough to numb the skin (a minute or two at most). Play around with locations; sometimes your thigh or hip might be less painful than your lower abdomen (or vice versa), and by all means, rotate locations from day to day!

**A word to the wise:** | Take the time to properly prepare for an injection of progesterone in oil. Heating the oil, icing your rear end, and lying down for the injection make it much less painful. Using a heating pad afterward can really reduce bruising and lumpiness. Many women who don't know these tricks wind up with large, very sore bruises and lumps where they did the injection. This can get problematic when you are doing them daily for weeks on end and you run out of nonbruised or pain-free spots to do the injection. This is not an injection that can be rotated to other body parts like your thigh (not if you ever want to walk again) so you need to take care of your derriere.

really need a lot of icing, this is one that does need a good cold spot), and afterward I recommend you lie or sit on a warm heating pad (I use a Band-Aid to mark the injection site to make sure that I get the right spot heated) for about fifteen minutes. This will minimize bruising and lumping. One thing to keep in mind about injecting progesterone is that it is a thick oil substance and will take much longer to inject than something like Pergonal or HCG. Be patient when you are first learning to do this injection. You will do so many of them that you will get the swing of it.

Sub-Q injections are much easier. You have many more places on your body to do them, and the needle is much smaller so it hurts less. You should be able to do a sub-Q injection by yourself, but by all means have someone else do it if you need to. One drawback to sub-Q injections is that the needle gauge is smaller, so the injection goes more slowly. Needle gauge is a funny thing; the higher the number, the smaller the gauge. A higher-gauge needle is thinner and has a smaller hole through which the medication is injected (that's why it's slower). Generally speaking, the higher the needle gauge, the less pain you'll have during an injection because the needle is getting thinner and thinner (smaller puncture wound). An IM injection uses a 22-gauge 1.5-inch needle. A typical sub-Q injection uses a 27.5-gauge half-inch needle. They come smaller than this (30 gauge, for example) if you need to minimize pain even more. Most people don't feel a 27.5-gauge needle stick, so don't worry if this is what your doctor prescribes. Take a look at the Appendix for more tips and specifics on preparing your injections.

Your doctor's office probably isn't going to write you a prescription for your stims and send you on your way with lots of needles you don't know how to use. Most clinics and doctors' offices offer patients training programs.

## Side Effects

Because your body is producing more hormones than usual and is subject to high-powered drugs, you may experience some side effects. Clomid can cause mood swings and breast tenderness. Many women, however, don't notice any side effects on Clomid. The more high-powered injectable stims like Pergonal, Gonal-F, and Follistim cause mood swings, breast tenderness, headaches, acne, bloating, and increased production of cervical fluid. Some of this is caused by the ovaries as they enlarge and multiple follicles develop (the abdominal bloating, for example). Other side effects are caused by increased E2 levels (breast tenderness and increased cervical fluid). Most women experience some side effects on stims.

Some of the drugs cause temporary side effects. There might, for example, be some tenderness or stinging at the injection site, especially with the IM injections. Follistim—although a sub-Q injection—is famous for its sting as it is injected and is nicknamed *FolliSTING*. Follistim is an excellent medication for some women, and there are ways to reduce the sting. I personally found this injection unbearable and switched to a different drug as soon as I could.

As you read this, you may not be able to fathom how you could possibly handle a self-administered injection or are worrying about bloating and migraine side effects. Trust me, if it gets you a baby—and even

**A word to the wise:** | There are ways to reduce the pain during and after an injection. With some of the drugs, FolliSTING in particular, you can try preparing the syringe and then letting it rest (sitting on a sterile countertop) for about fifteen minutes. Often this reduces the sting from the drug as it enters body tissue. You can also try icing the injection site for a few minutes before administering the medication. This often reduces any pain from the needle stick and can numb the area to any stinging or burning from the drug as it is injected. You can also ask your clinic about changing needle sizes. I found that on very painful injections it helped to use a smaller-gauge needle. On one injection I used a 30-gauge needle. With this small a needle, it took longer to inject the medication, but there was less of a sting from the drug. Some women find certain areas of the body more sensitive. If your lower abdomen is a painful place to inject, try your thigh or the fleshy part of your outer hip. Try these tips by themselves or in combination to help ease any pain you may experience from these injections.

if it doesn't—it's worth it. And it's really not so bad once you get going. (Just think about the size needle they use for epidurals! Now that's something to look forward to.)

## Going in for Training

**What it is:** Most REs' offices teach you everything you need to know to get through a cycle (so you—as I did—can forget about it all just in time for your first injection).

**What's involved:** Whether it is one-on-one training with a nurse or a group seminar, I strongly encourage you to go with your husband or partner.

**A word to the wise:** | Having a cycle buddy can be very important. Not only will having someone to talk to about how you are feeling and what's going on during your cycle reassure you, but having this person in your life will help diminish the feelings of isolation that infertility treatment can cause. There are some downsides, however, so choose your cycle buddy carefully. First, not everyone is going to get pregnant from her cycle. How will you or your cycle buddy react if one of you gets pregnant and the other doesn't? Or how will it be between you if you both get pregnant but one of you miscarries? I know these seem like grim things to think about, but knowing that these are possibilities and talking about them beforehand with your cycle buddy, or even avoiding a cycle buddy who seems very competitive or unsupportive, can spare you a lot of grief at the end of the cycle. You want a cycle buddy who thinks like you do and who is supportive and nurturing. You want a cycle buddy who is encouraging and gets you thinking about silver linings and the good side of things when things seem overwhelming and hard. If you find someone like this to help you though the cycle, you will be ahead of the game.

The nurse will provide a step-by-step guide to injection. If it's a group training seminar, you'll have the opportunity to meet other patients who will be cycling around the same time as you. This may make you feel less alone, and you may even meet a cycle buddy this way. Attending training also is a great way to develop a more personal relationship with one of the nurses in your doctor's office or clinic, someone who you'll feel more comfortable calling with questions or problems.

Lastly, the notes you take and the information you get during training can prove to be invaluable. Charlie and I got a videotape of a woman administering an injection; it showed everything, from syringe preparation to Band-Aid administration afterward. I can't tell you how many times we watched that video the night we had to do my very first injection.

Boy did having that video relieve a lot of stress! The video or my notes from our training session answered every question we had! In case you need it or have questions, I put step-by-step instructions on how to administer an injection in the Appendix at the back of the book.

# 12

# Beginning Your Infertility Treatment

## IT'S EXCITING FOR ABOUT A DAY

You have decided on a treatment plan (IUI, IVF, donor egg), gone in for training, picked up your stims, and are getting really anxious (and excited, too)! Or perhaps you're still trying to decide what treatment option is best for you and want to know more about what life is like during an IUI/IVF cycle. This chapter provides a day-to-day description of a prototypical cycle. It will give you an idea of what you'll be doing and will also provide some tips about ways to make your cycle easier.

## Getting Going

The first thing you'll do is schedule your cycle. Sounds like a no-brainer, doesn't it (gee, I think I could have figured that out for myself!). Well, it's not. First, you need to find out what your clinic or doctor's office requires before you can begin. You may have to go in for blood work on cycle day 3 (CD3) to ensure that your hormone levels are within normal ranges for treatment. You may have already done this and may resent doing it again, but remember, these levels fluctuate. If certain hormone levels were high before and are lower now, it could be an indication that this is a great time for you to cycle. (I'll talk more about CD3 blood work later in this chapter.) You may need additional blood work again in a couple of weeks (around or after the time of ovulation) or close to the beginning of your cycle to confirm that it's safe to start medication. Make sure you find out when and if you need to have any preliminary blood tests.

Your clinic may also have some financial hoops for you to jump through. Even if they don't want to run a credit check (yes, some places do this), you may want to talk to their billing or patient services department to make sure you're fully aware of the charges you'll incur and whether or not there are financial services available (like the shared risk or guarantee programs discussed in chapter 9) that may help you manage the cost of treatment. Don't underestimate your clinic's ability to surprise you with unexpected costs. I didn't know pregnancy tests weren't included in the cost of an IVF cycle, and after seven of them (at $300 a pop), my bankbook got dangerously low. Trust me, it really makes sense to sit down and go over this stuff with the patient services or billing department.

Once you have taken care of the money planning, it's time to figure out when to actually do your cycle. First, take a look at your menstrual calendar and figure out when your next few cycles are. Scheduling cycles for IUI patients generally isn't a problem. But for IVF patients, scheduling can be more difficult.

There are three things to keep in mind when you are scheduling an IVF cycle. They are: (1) your RE's or clinic's calendar (IVF patients have somewhat limited windows of time in which to cycle as we will discuss in a moment), (2) your menstrual cycle, and (3) your work/stress level. Each will play a role in determining how soon you will be able to start an IVF cycle.

IUI patients need only consider their work/stress schedule and menstrual cycle (most clinics cycle IUI patients year round). If you're undergoing IVF, your clinic or RE's office probably has blocks of time every few months when it is closed for embryology lab cleaning (it must be scrupulously clean at all times to prevent the embryos from contracting

**A word to the wise:** | Whether you're doing IVF or IUI, you want to make sure that the weeks surrounding your cycle are as relaxed as possible. You probably won't be feeling well for portions of your cycle, and you want to be able to take time to take care of yourself. Believe me, you don't want to be exerting yourself after insemination or embryo transfer; you will need and want time to rest. More importantly, however, your cycle is likely to be more successful if you're relaxed.

viruses and being contaminated with bacteria). Most fertility centers break their calendars into four "series" or "cycles" each year (the number varies from clinic to clinic). Each series lasts about two and a half months and allows the clinic to schedule patients around the lab's cleaning schedule. Generally, your clinic will have someone responsible for scheduling IVF patients into each series (you will want to know who this person is as soon as you decide to do IVF). This person—generally called something like "patient coordinator"—juggles the series calendar with the number of patients cycling at any given time.

Because each series can accommodate only a certain number of patients, you may not be able to get into the next series on the calendar. (Doesn't this just suck!) Sometimes you have to wait a few months to cycle in a series that still has reservations available. (Aargh!) There may be a wait list, so make sure to have your name put on it in case someone cancels their reservation.

When scheduling an IVF cycle within a series, your menstrual cycle has to be timed within that series. Each series has two dates you'll need to pay attention to; in order to qualify, you must get your period after the date the series begins but before the last date when the series is closing. Depending on your medication protocol (down regulation or flare), if the series starts at the beginning of April but your April period won't start until the end of that month, you won't be starting your stims until the middle of May. Your clinic will make your reservation based on the *date that you're expected to start stims.*

The next thing you need to consider is what is likely to be going on in your life when you want to cycle. If there is anything likely to cause excess stress or place large demands on your time and energy during your cycle, you might want to consider cycling at a different time or rescheduling other priorities. It is very, very difficult to balance the demands of infertility treatment with a high-stress, fast-paced job.

It is especially important to make sure you have plenty of time to rest during an IVF cycle, as IVF cycles are physically demanding. Even if you've already done an IUI cycle or three and think you can handle it, think again. Your ovaries will produce many more eggs, and you'll take stronger drugs to make this happen. The stims phase will be more intense during IVF; two additional procedures are involved. First you'll have oocyte retrieval (this is the egg retrieval and is commonly known just as "retrieval"). This is a surgical procedure, so you'll be anesthetized while your eggs are removed from your ovaries. After retrieval you'll have embryo transfer ("transfer"). Transfer generally doesn't involve anesthesia, but you may receive a mild sedative (I talk in detail about these procedures later in this chapter), and you'll need time to recuperate in a recovery room. In contrast, IUI cycles require one fairly easy insemination, which doesn't hurt, involve anesthesia, or require recuperation periods. After insemination and embryo transfer, you'll need to take it easy for a few days. In IVF programs, women are usually put on modified bed rest for a few days after embryo transfer and asked to take it very easy until their pregnancy test (almost two weeks later).

Make sure that your work schedule can accommodate these demands or that you can take vacation or sick leave when needed, and that you will not be under undue pressure while managing all of this. I recommend that you take time off from work during the entire IVF cycle. This may seem impossible, and you may have to tell your employer that you're having some sort of medical treatment (and even go on disability), but you'll find the cycle is much easier if you aren't worried about getting in to work on time after daily monitoring, making a meeting when you need to do an injection, or worrying that you are cramping and spotting after transfer and should be resting when you need to get to a meeting. IUI and IVF cycles are stressful enough; piling on work pressure may result in your losing your mind and jeopardizing your cycle outcome. Don't underestimate the way stress affects your cycle.

Recent research shows that women who are more relaxed and who receive adequate emotional support during IUI and IVF cycles have better pregnancy and live-birth rates. I talk a lot about the importance of managing stress later on in the chapter, but for right now, as you plan your cycle, think hard about coordinating your cycle and schedule so as to eliminate as much pressure as possible and thus increase your chances of success.

## Creating a Care Package

Once you've organized the timing, start thinking about ways to nurture yourself during the cycle. My good friend Ann (my first cycle buddy) had already done IVF twice when we first met. One of the wisest things she told me was to make my cycle a special time and fill it with things to pamper and distract me.

With Ann's help, I created a care package I could use when facing a tough day or moment in my cycle. All women undergoing any sort of infertility treatment should have a care package on hand to remind them that they're important and need to take care of themselves. Believe it or not, it's easy to forget about *you* during your cycle as everyone starts focusing on your follicle development, E2 levels, and embryo quality. A care package will remind you that you deserve to be treated well during this process. *You* matter!

Ann and I went shopping for face masks, scented moisturizers and shower gels, books, magazines, meditation tapes, and scented candles. I made a list of videos (mostly chick flicks) I wanted to rent and started a new knitting project, a sweater for me (not a gift or something for a baby). I got a makeover at my favorite department store and bought new makeup for my care package. When my mother and Charlie asked me what they could do to help, I told them to get me gift certificates for manicures, pedicures, and massages. I also stocked up on manicure supplies so I could do my own when I didn't feel well enough to go out. I got my hair cut, colored, and highlighted before the cycle started so that I wouldn't have to worry about hair dye affecting egg quality or a growing embryo (not that it would necessarily, I just tend to worry about things like this). Lastly, I went shopping for a special box to put everything in. Before my cycle started, I put all my supplies in the box and put it on a shelf in my closet.

Shopping for the care package was tremendously soothing and provided a productive activity during the days I was waiting for my baby-making injections to start. It was a great way to divert my anxiety and fear. You don't have to spend a lot of money on your care package. I budgeted carefully and spent money on the things I really wanted (like meditation tapes). You can borrow books from the library if you don't want to incur the cost of buying them, and you can find great deals at dollar stores, drugstores, and outlets. Many video stores offer coupon books, as do candle and bath and body stores. I saved several of my regular monthly subscription magazines and put them in the care package box before I read them; that way I only bought a few new magazines. You don't have to go hog wild here, just try to set aside a few things that will cheer you up on tough days when you find yourself feeling bloated, ugly, hormonal, and depressed.

## Living Through the Cycle

Whether you're an IUIer or IVFer, this is going to be a long, hard month. (Although there are some differences, this section is written generically for both IUI and IVF.) IVF patients will feel more uncomfortable than IUI patients, and they'll have more procedures. If you've done IUIs before and are moving on to IVF, remember you shouldn't expect it to feel the same. But the day-to-day routine is pretty similar. The experiences I describe are based on my four ovulation inductions for IUIs, five and a half IVF cycles (I had one cycle that was canceled mid–stims phase), and the experience of my friends.

The basic rule is: the more sensitive your body is, the more you'll feel. If you usually don't feel anything when you ovulate, you might not notice when your ovaries begin to enlarge and you start to produce multiple follicles. If, however, you are like me and have a very sensitive body and *feel* when you ovulate (it's called Mittelschmerz, or midcycle pain), stims may not be so much fun. Don't worry if you don't feel anything, ever. Some women make a ton of eggs and don't feel anything at all. If you're concerned about how comfortable or uncomfortable you should be, call your clinic or IVF nurse.

If you're doing an IUI cycle, chances are your medication dosage is much lower than that of the IVF woman (lucky you!). Aside from minor mood swings or breast tenderness, you might not feel anything but minor discomfort from the injections. Women with sensitive ovaries may experience twinges and pressure as follicles develop. You may also experience mild bloating (like you get before your period) and constipation. If you experience sharp pain or severe bloating, call your doctor's office right away so they can make sure that you're okay.

Let me tell you, even after five and half IVF cycles, I am shocked at how uncomfortable I get. In the beginning you may feel only a little soreness at the injection site and maybe a tiny twinge in your lower abdomen. But after a few days, as your ovaries are kicking into high gear, you may feel crampy, bloated, tired, and constipated. You may also have some sharp pains (I think it feels like having little butter knives or tiny rocks poking at my ovaries), breast tenderness, and/or major mood swings.

For both IUI and IVF patients, after about a week on stims, if you're responding well to the drugs and/or have a reasonably sensitive body, you *will* feel those ovaries and you *will* be tired! A week after I start stims (seven nights of injections), I'm very bloated (jeans are uncomfortable unless they are baggy) and crampy. I also get very tired and a little bit bitchy. Getting up in the morning for monitoring is a major drag (please let me sleep!) and I pop Tylenol about as frequently as the bottle tells me it is safe. (I can feel when it wears off, how sucky is that?) The ultrasounds start getting uncomfortable, too, and more than once I have asked the doctor scanning me to be *very* gentle.

At the very end, I can feel my ovaries, even with Tylenol, and I can't wait to get insemination, or retrieval, over with. My mood swings are intense, and during some cycles I cry for little or no reason every day. The bloating is obvious, too, and I start wearing big shirts over baggy pants. I even look a little pregnant. Dr. Chung once explained that (during an IVF cycle) my ovaries get to be the size of small oranges as they enlarge with the follicles. Once you take your HCG trigger injection, however, you'll feel a little better.

You might also be moody and strung out from the stress of managing your cycle. Though it's totally normal to be stressed out from what you're going through (I would be surprised if you weren't), stress is counterproductive. Lowering your stress level may increase your chances of getting pregnant, so don't neglect your state of mind.

Okay, let's start the blow-by-blow of a typical cycle.

**EVERYTHING UP TO AND INCLUDING THE DAY OF YOUR HCG TRIGGER INJECTION**
Beginning on CD3 (it may be CD2 for you if you're on a flare protocol) you go in for blood work and ultrasound monitoring; this day marks the beginning of your stims phase. Your E2 level should be below 50 and your LH level less than 5 (these values may be a little different at your clinic). Some clinics may also check your P4 (progesterone); this should be less than 2. If any of these values are higher than normal, you will be asked to continue your Lupron for a few days and come back for repeat testing. If you're doing a flare protocol or an IUI—where you have not yet been suppressed or will not be suppressed—your doctor is also looking to see that your FSH is less than 10 (again this number varies from clinic to clinic; some clinics will let you cycle with an FSH as high as 20).

On your first day of monitoring, CD3, you'll also have an ultrasound.

You want your ovaries to be free of cysts and your uterine environment to appear normal with a lining less than 5 mm. A nurse will call with your instructions for starting your stims that night and tell you when to come back for your next round with the vampires (more blood work). Some of the bigger IVF centers may keep patients on Lupron for a few extra days to stagger them and avoid having too many patients going to retrieval on the same day.

Assuming all is normal, you will give yourself your first injection(s) of stims (expect to freak out a little) and then have a day to recuperate (repeating your injection the next night, of course) before going back to the clinic. You will go in every other morning in the beginning for blood work and probably follow this pattern until CD7 or CD9, when you'll start going in every day for blood work and ultrasounds.

It starts getting tiring now. The morning monitoring really takes it out of you. You also start to feel uncomfortable now and very emotional. The wait for the afternoon phone call is excruciating, especially if there is a question you want answered. You will need your care package, and you'll need your friends and family members to be very helpful and supportive. Your partner should be helping you around the house and giving you time to rest. If, during the course of the day, all you can do is get to the office and home, that's a major accomplishment. And don't worry if the urge to cry takes over at extremely inopportune moments. Have a good cry and learn to take each day one minute at a time.

But it also starts to get exciting now. Your follicles start to grow day by day; it's pretty amazing to go in one morning and have them all measure 11.5 mm and find the following day they're all 13.5 mm. If you were particularly uncomfortable during the night it can be validating to see the growth in follicle size. You may get your HCG prescription (remember to get it filled right away, even if you won't need it for a day or so!), and you may start thinking about when your insemination or retrieval is going to be.

## MONITORING: HOW'S MY CYCLE PROGRESSING?

I know you're going to obsess about how your cycle is progressing (it's normal), so let me give you some tips that'll keep things in perspective during the stims phase. As you'll see (or may already know), daily monitoring during the stims phase can drive even the sanest of us over the edge.

**Don't Have Any Expectations.** Every woman's cycle is unique. Stop having expectations right now! Each woman responds differently to meds; the same woman on the same meds may respond differently in each cycle. None of my IUI or five-plus IVF cycles was ever remotely similar. Each cycle presents a new set of issues. I never know what to expect, so I don't expect. Let the cycle unfold day by day, and you'll be much happier.

Don't (please don't) compare yourself to people you know who've gone through this or anyone who may sit next to you in the waiting room at your clinic or doctor's office. It's very tempting, but don't get sucked into this game. Don't compare what your E2 level is and how many follicles you have with what your friend did in the cycle where she got pregnant or what the woman sitting next to you in the waiting room is experiencing.

**It's How *Your* Body Responds to the Meds That's Important!** I know you're wondering and worrying about how you should be responding to your stims. Because every woman is so different, it's really hard to specify what *you* should be doing. Let your cycle evolve, and let your RE earn her money managing your cycle as it does. You need to be very patient with your body and RE.

You will start on a certain dosage of stims and, depending on your E2 level (how fast it is rising and how high it is) and how your follicles are developing (as monitored by ultrasound), you'll gradually reduce the dosage. For some women it can take several days before the dosage is lowered. By reducing the dosage, your RE is telling your body to stop producing new follicles and instead focus on growing and developing the follicles you already have. If you aren't developing many follicles, your doctor might increase your stims dose. More likely, however, she'll keep you on the initial dose and patiently wait for follicles to appear. Eventually, when you start producing follicles and your E2 level has risen to an appropriate level, you will start to cut back the meds. Again, there are different protocols, so if you're told something different, don't worry.

Your RE will base her decisions about your evening stims dose on your E2 level that morning, which measures the amount of estrogen (estradiol) your body is producing as follicles develop. Rising levels indicate follicles are growing in your ovaries. You want the E2 level to rise between blood tests; how much it rises depends on many, many things. Don't focus on it too much, or it'll drive you crazy! As long as it's rising steadily, you can relax. If it rises slowly at first, this isn't necessarily a cause for concern, nor is a rapid rise at the end. Let your doctor worry about how high your level is getting or how slowly it is rising.

That said, too high an E2 level puts you at risk for ovarian hyperstimulation syndrome (OHSS), which is a potentially life-threatening condition (discussed in detail in chapter 7), that can occur during the stims phase or after retrieval and transfer has taken place. What is "too high" an E2 level during the stims phase will depend on your clinic's judgment and how many follicles you're developing (some clinics will cancel patients with E2 levels in the 3,000 range, while others will allow patients to cycle up to 5,000). I started to hyperstimulate once during stims, and it wasn't fun.

If your E2 level is very high and your RE is concerned you might hyperstimulate, your RE can "coast" you for a day or two in an attempt to rescue your cycle. However, your follicles must be at least 14 to 15 mm in size in order to be coasted. If you coast, you'll get very little or no medication (you'll continue taking Lupron to stay suppressed so you don't ovulate on your own) so your body continues to produce eggs without elevating your E2 to dangerous levels. You want the E2 level to rise a little bit while coasting or even plateau; it's also okay if it drops slightly. You don't want your E2 level to crash; to drop, for example, from 4,600 to 1,200 in a twenty-four hour period. If your E2 level starts to crash, you may have poor egg quality. Your doctor will probably cancel your cycle (this is what happened to me). If your E2 keeps rising (but more slowly) or remains stable while you're coasting, that means your body is still working on potentially good eggs. Decisions about canceling your cycle because of OHSS are complex. Talk to your doctor about what she thinks is in your best interest.

If your cycle is canceled, remember that your doctor is concerned with both getting you pregnant *and* keeping you healthy. OHSS really can be life threatening. Sometimes it truly is better to be safe than sorry. Console yourself with the knowledge that women who hyperstimulate or are at risk for hyperstimulation—including those who've been coasted—have higher than average pregnancy rates.

Low E2 levels can signify immature or unhealthy eggs. But there's no need to panic if you've cycled before and are suddenly having a cycle with much lower E2 levels. Many times, however, low E2 levels indicate a lack of follicular development and may result in your cycle being converted from IVF to IUI or canceled completely. It will depend on how many follicles you're making. Some women will be allowed to go to retrieval with very few eggs. Most IVF patients, however, need at least four or five good follicles to be candidates for retrieval. It can be devastating when an IVF cycle is converted to IUI or canceled. Don't be afraid to talk to your doctor about why she's converting or canceling your cycle. There are some instances where your doctor will proceed to retrieval after you've discussed the risks.

You may also be wondering what the perfect E2 level is. *There isn't one.* It varies from woman to woman and depends on how many follicles you've got. The rule of thumb is that for every mature follicle, your E2 level should be between 100 and 200 p/ml (parts per milliliter). This is true for both IUI and IVF patients. But this is really just a gauge; only your doctor can judge when your E2 level is at an "ideal" level. However, one indication that your eggs are nearing maturation is when your E2 level plateaus, and there is a very small rise between two of your morning blood tests.

Again, don't worry too much about your E2 level. If you focus on every aspect of infertility treatment (*most of it is out of your control*), you'll drive yourself insane. If you make it to retrieval, you've passed the first big IVF hurdle! When you get your trigger injection of HCG for insemination, you're thirty-six hours away from having your partner's sperm inside you doing their thing. This is exciting stuff!

Your RE—of course—doesn't look solely at your E2 level as a measure of your progress toward retrieval or insemination. She also looks at the development of your follicles on ultrasound. Sadly, counting follicles can become just as obsessive as monitoring your E2 level on a daily basis. This brings us to my next tip.

**Focus on Quality of Eggs, not Quantity.** Quality not quantity: that's your mantra for the cycle. All right, I know you want the inside scoop; how many eggs does your RE want to see during an IUI/IVF cycle? Mantra aside, here's the deal.

IUI patients probably need about three follicles. This number provides you the best chance of getting pregnant, with a reasonable risk of conceiving multiples. Any more follicles, and your doctor may be concerned about you winding up with a high-order multiple pregnancy (triplets or greater), and it may lead her to suggest converting you from IUI to IVF. Going to IVF instead of IUI may help minimize the risk of a multiple conception (I had a friend who did this and got pregnant). I had five eggs one IUI cycle and had to promise, swear, and practically sign in blood that I would selectively reduce a high-order multiple pregnancy (in other words, terminate one or more of the pregnancies) before she would allow me to go through with the insemination.

If you only have one follicle with an IUI, this is not a horrible failure. It only takes one egg to get pregnant, and you have to remember that this is probably a very healthy egg. Plus, the sperm is going to be placed in an optimal location to meet your egg. While you're freaking out about only having one egg (most of us would be a little disappointed), try to keep in mind that at some centers one good egg per IUI cycle is thought ideal.

IVF patients want a significantly higher number of follicles than IUI patients. Not every egg will be mature and/or fertilize, so the more you have, the better your chances. But too many eggs can be a problem. I know you've heard stories of women producing eighteen, twenty-eight, or even more eggs with an IVF cycle. When IVF first started, doctors believed that a large quantity of eggs provided the best chance of conception.

Doctors now realize, however, that egg quality is as important, if not more important, than egg quantity (hence my mantra). Generally speaking, lots of eggs aren't the greatest thing in IVF-land. It is likely that not all of those eggs are healthy. It's not uncommon to wind up with only four healthy embryos when you started out with twenty eggs. Very few women produce huge numbers of healthy eggs. If you're one of the women who produce twenty amazingly healthy eggs, my ovaries and I salute you! Chances are, however, this isn't going to be you and I don't want you to be upset about it. Most clinics feel that recruitment of ten to twelve eggs for IVF produces the greatest likelihood of success.

There you have it, the scoop on egg quantity for IUI/IVF. Notwithstanding this information (and the obsession it will surely bring), I want you to focus on your mantra and on my next tip (maybe make it another mantra).

**Slow and Steady Wins the Race!** If you're an IVF patient, you also want to ignore how long it takes for your eggs to mature. Some women will stimulate and make follicles very quickly, but most women take about two weeks to get to retrieval. IUI patients frequently take stims for shorter periods than IVF patients do, but it can feel like forever for you, too. The longer it takes, the harder it is. But remember that every day you think you can't take it anymore is another day spent making good quality eggs. You will really need patience and perseverance to get through this.

In addition to growing slowly, you want your follicles to grow at roughly the same rate. (Basically, you want them all to be roughly the same size each day they are measured.) If there is too big a gap in follicle size, you might be at risk for developing a lead follicle. If this happens, your body may stop investing energy in the smaller follicles and may devote energy to the big one. This is okay for IUI patients but not good news for IVFers. What starts out as a good cycle produces just one egg.

**A word to the wise:** | You want to make sure you get your prescription for HCG filled ahead of time. This prescription cannot be called in to your pharmacy; a doctor must handwrite the form in triplicate, and if you don't have it the night you need it you're going to have to do some serious scrambling to get it filled at the last minute. This is also a time-sensitive injection because your retrieval or insemination time is specifically calculated based on when you got your HCG trigger injection, so screwing up the timing because you can't fill the prescription is going to pose some major problems for your clinic.

There is nothing you can do about this. If it happens, you can still do an IUI, but IVF is probably out of the question.

Assuming that a lead follicle isn't developing, some variability in rate of growth is okay. This is why you should let your doctor worry about follicle size and rate of growth. As long as each follicle grows every day, even if they aren't all the "right" size, everything should be fine. This is one of those issues you can and *should* let your doctor sweat out while you kick back and focus on success!

Mature follicles generally measure in the 18 mm range or larger (I have gotten mature eggs out of much smaller follicles). Once you reach this point (with a corresponding E2 level for mature follicles), you'll get your HCG trigger injection. (This is the hormone your body makes when it's pregnant, so if you take a home pregnancy test within a week to ten days after taking this injection, it will give you a false positive result.) HCG tells the ovaries to finish ripening your eggs and get them ready for fertilization. Your doctor will determine the best day for you to receive HCG.

By the way, I have no idea how doctors figure out when to give patients HCG. There seems to be such a variance in E2 levels and follicle sizes. You pay your doctor the big bucks, and if you ask me, this is one of the times she earns them.

The day after your HCG injection most clinics have you come in for blood work. Your LH level the next day will confirm that you actually injected HCG. Believe it or not, some patients don't mix the HCG properly and either wind up injecting the dilutent without having mixed the medication in (so they are injecting sterile water) or they inject the wrong amount of HCG. In addition to checking your LH level, your RE will check your E2 level to confirm that your HCG was timed properly in relation to the maturation of your eggs. You want your E2 level to go up (even just a little bit) after you receive your HCG as this means your eggs are continuing to grow and mature. If your E2 level drops more than 20 percent, your doctor knows that you received the HCG too late (even the most skilled and experienced REs sometimes misjudge the delicate timing for administration of HCG). You may still be able to do an insemination or have retrieval, but your egg quality may be compromised.

Your RE will also be checking your uterine lining during all those ultrasounds (one more thing to obsess about, how great is that!). You want to have a nice thick lining for those embryos. A lining of 8 to 9 mm or thicker is considered healthy enough for implantation. Linings of 18 mm have been reported, but excessive thickness—in the absence of abnormalities—should not hinder implantation.

Your uterine lining should also be triple stripe, meaning that there is a specific pattern of development, usually characterized by three stripes (top, middle, and bottom is one simplified way to describe it). The layers should be uniform in size and placement. If, for example, you have an uneven stripe down the middle, that could indicate a uterine polyp or other abnormality that's interfering with the development of the lining. Some abnormalities don't interfere with implantation. If your doctor is concerned about your lining, talk to her and see what she feels is best. If you're doing IVF, you always have the option of freezing your embryos and removing the abnormality surgically or waiting to see if it resolves on its own. Similarly, if your lining isn't developing well and is too thin, it can be treated in a subsequent cycle using supplemental estrogen or even Viagra (this is a new treatment and is somewhat controversial).

**Pace Yourself.** Getting to the end of the stims phase is tough. Despite my cautionary words, you've been worrying and obsessing about how your cycle is progressing. You are going to your doctor's office or clinic every other day and then, eventually, every day for blood work and ultrasound. Depending on how busy the office is, you can spend up to two hours a morning getting through monitoring. You're lucky if your clinic can get you in and out in under an hour when you need to have both blood work and an ultrasound done. Mine *never* could. Combine the stress of watching E2 levels rise and follicles grow with the time-consuming nature of the monitoring, and you need to be prepared to be very tired and strung out. Basically, you're tired from daily monitoring, exhausted from the hormonal and physical roller coaster you're on, uncomfortable from your enlarged ovaries, and sore from multiple injections. It's *not* fun!

This is a long haul; you need to pace yourself. Take it a day at a time, an hour at a time, a minute at a time. Pull out your care package and find something nurturing and cheery. Take a long, warm shower and a nap. Eat good, hearty protein-packed meals. Your clinic may have instructed you to stop exercising. If you haven't listened to them, *now* is the time to stop exercising; stop feeling guilty about not exercising when you have this huge pooched belly. Sit-ups are not going to make it go away anyway, so why bother torturing yourself? Above all else, keep your strength up. If you need to cry every day, *go ahead!* If you have crying jags that last for days, *that's okay!* There may be more hurdles (okay, there are definitely more hurdles) ahead, so take it easy, and let your husband or partner baby you as much as possible.

## MANAGING STRESS

The October 2001 issue of *Fertility and Sterility* reported that the most stressed-out group of women undergoing infertility treatment were 93 percent *less* likely to have a baby than the more relaxed patients. The experience is bad enough, the treatment makes it even more stressful, and that makes you even less likely to have a baby! What are you supposed to do? Can you really control your stress in order to improve your chance of conceiving? Yes, you can.

This is hard for all of us. Research shows that infertility causes emotional responses similar to that experienced by patients with cancer and long-term serious diseases. This is a crisis; denying it is just going to make you feel more isolated, depressed, and scared. Accepting your feelings is important, but it isn't going to make you feel better overnight. You need to take proactive steps to manage your stress.

Let me now sing the praises of meditation. Lying quietly and visualizing images that are relaxing and soothing can be very helpful. If you're inexperienced with meditation, start with small increments of time (it takes time to get good at being still and quieting your mind) and imagine yourself on a beach in the warm sun, sitting by a smooth lake, or standing in the middle of a beautiful mountain field. Focus on the image and try and get it as specific and detailed as possible.

As you get familiar with the experience of visualization, you can use it to help your cycle progress and may feel more empowered. Sometimes I would try to stimulate my ovaries by imagining showers of white light raining down and energizing them. This may sound far out to you, but it really helped me feel in control of and connected to my body.

If this doesn't work for you, try guided meditation tapes. Many clinics offer these for free, or you can find them at a local bookstore, wellness center, or on the Web. I have listed some books and places to go for more information on working with meditation in the Resources section at the back of the book. Don't overlook relaxation therapy, meditation, or visualization. Research with cancer patients and infertile women consistently shows that this stuff boosts the immune system, lowers levels of stress-related chemicals in the brain, and increases the success rates of treatment.

Hypnosis also can be effective. There are therapists (who even take insurance) trained in helping you deal with complex issues through hypnosis. There are also lots of books on self-hypnosis that are helpful. Hypnosis is even being used effectively for pain management in childbirth.

Acupuncture, massage, and yoga also work to manage stress. Even though I'm petrified of needles, I got such a rush and felt so balanced after my acupuncture sessions that it was worth the anxiety over the needles. Acupuncture is based on the idea that there are specific energy meridians (points) in the body that, when stimulated, can help you relax and heal. I believe it because it worked for me.

I also found it relaxing to lie down on the acupuncturist's table and often used this time for meditation and visualization. Sometimes I just fell asleep. A study reported in the April 2002 *Fertility and Sterility* confirmed that patients undergoing acupuncture during IVF cycles have almost twice the success rates (42.5 percent compared to 26.3 percent) of patients who don't undergo the therapy. The researchers urged more studies to help medical science better understand how acupuncture works. Sometimes what seems far out really works!

Massage is great because it physically relaxes your muscles and helps release stress-building toxins from body tissue. Touch has long been known to have healing effects, and there is something very soothing about spending an hour lying on a table while someone ministers to your poor aching body. If you can't afford a professional massage, borrow a book from the library and have your husband or partner give you a nice long back rub. There are also ways to massage yourself that can be very relaxing.

Lastly, yoga is a great mind/body stress management tool. I am not talking about power yoga—the type of yoga practiced by Madonna and Sting—but yoga that focuses on breath, movement, and stretching. If you're into yoga or willing to explore it, find a class that focuses on body alignment and harmonizing energy and breath. These are the least difficult from an exercise standpoint (although you still get a good workout) and impart the greatest benefit to your mood. If you are like me and hate exercising in a group, there are some great yoga videotapes worth renting and buying. You don't need much in the way of equipment (a towel and a folded blanket are generally enough to get you started) or space in your living room. If you like taking classes, check out the yoga studios in your area. I was surprised to find that many of them offered classes for women undergoing fertility treatment. Some IVF centers even offer yoga classes to their patients.

Reading, watching television, or going to the movies can also help manage stress. Remember that the most effective stress management tools are those that help you retrain your brain to think in more positive life- and self-affirming ways. If you would rather read than take a yoga class or meditate, maybe take a walk through the self-help section at your library or bookstore and see if you can find a book that not only distracts you from treatment but also helps you look at life differently. Talking can be a big help, either with other infertility patients in an organized group session or in one-on-one therapy. You may benefit from therapy with someone trained in dealing with infertility; you can find people like this through RESOLVE or the American Infertility Association (see the Re- sources section for contact information). Or just find a therapist you like. I have friends who swear by infertility support groups; there are also pregnancy loss support groups, and couples groups.

Whatever stress-reduction tool you choose, the goal is to find ways to feel calmer and more in control of your body and life, more *empowered!* Try to think in positive terms about your infertility and about the fact that you *can* and *will* become a mother!

## IUI PATIENTS: EVERYTHING FROM INSEMINATION TO FERTILIZATION

By this point you're feeling better because you've made it through the stims phase and are looking forward to moving on to the two-week wait (when you're waiting to find out if you're pregnant). You are also feeling better; something about the HCG trigger injection alleviates some of the discomfort you may have been experiencing.

The day of insemination is pretty low key. Despite your excitement, it's awkward leaving your hubby to make his "contribution" and then waiting while his sample is prepared (this can be over an hour). When you get your husband's sample back, you'll pore over the analysis to see how much sperm you have to fertilize your egg(s).

If the sample quantity increases after it is prepared, this does *not* mean you have more sperm. Rather, it means that the concentration of sperm per fluid volume has increased. Try not to obsess about the number of sperm. All it takes is one, and the sperm you're getting from the andrology lab (the people who work with sperm) have had all sorts of fun things done to them so they can better achieve fertilization. Your chance at conception is much better than it ever is after sex.

Once you get into the exam/procedure room, you may be surprised to discover the actual procedure is fairly low-tech. You may be given a hospital gown, but more likely you'll get a sheet and be told to undress from the waist down (fancy, eh?). You get up on a table, stick your feet in stirrups, and have that familiar meeting with a (hopefully warm) speculum. The doctor or nurse gently inserts a catheter through your cervix into the base of your uterine cavity, depresses a plunger attached to the syringe with the semen, and voilà, you're done!

Take nice, long, deep breaths, hold your husband's or partner's hand, and think nice thoughts about smiling babies. Sometimes there is some pinching and cramping from the catheter, but more often than not the procedure is completely painless. The catheter and speculum come out, and you lie on the table for twenty minutes or so and give the sperm a chance to do their job. Then you go home and go about your life for the next two weeks.

I recommend taking it easy for a few days, especially if you have any spotting. In the first couple of days after an IUI this spotting probably is from your cervix being irritated by the catheter; heavy bleeding should be reported to your doctor. Fertilization should take place in about twenty-four to thirty-six hours. Then it takes a few days for the fertilized zygote/embryo to roll and bump its way down your fallopian tube, into your uterus, and then another day or so for it to find a place to nestle and implant. Implantation takes place roughly five days after insemination (it can vary from woman to woman and embryo to embryo).

## IVF PATIENTS: EVERYTHING ABOUT RETRIEVAL

Retrieval is a surgical procedure that requires anesthesia. It's called retrieval because your eggs are surgically "retrieved" from your ovaries (it's also called harvesting). You can't eat or drink anything the night before and the morning of your surgery. You will be hungry and cranky, and this makes retrieval less exciting and fun. Retrieval also may be performed in a hospital (not necessarily at your clinic), which can increase your anxiety level. If you're particularly nervous or concerned about retrieval, talk to your doctor.

You'll be in an operating room or something similar. I don't know about you, but operating rooms freak me out. I think they're horribly intimidating, and they always seem to be freezing. (Why these rooms have subarctic temperatures I don't know; you'd think they'd keep them warm since you're naked!) It also means lots of scary instruments, bright lights, beeping machines, and people scurrying around you. If the environment scares you, try to breathe deeply and close your eyes. Don't be afraid to ask to hold a nurse's hand (I *have* to do this). Hopefully, you'll be put to sleep right away. But be prepared to be awake during the unpleasant and embarrassing surgical preparation where you're draped and painted (inside, *yuck,* and out) with a cold, antibacterial solution.

Either just before you're taken into the operating room for retrieval or while you're inside, your husband (assuming you're not using donor or frozen sperm) will be taken to facilities where he can "produce" his contribution to your IVF cycle. Men truly get off easily in IVF!

Retrieval can be a relatively quick twenty-minute procedure. Clinics that cycle many patients and do multiple retrievals every day (sometimes as many as fifteen per day) will have you in and out of the OR faster than you can imagine. Facilities that perform retrievals less frequently may take up to an hour or more. There are many medications that can be used to knock you out, but eggs and embryos are extremely fragile, and there are only a few anesthetics that don't harm eggs and embryos. Most common among the safe anesthetics—and what you're more than likely to get—is a drug called Propofol. In my book, Propofol qualifies as a good drug; it will have you out cold, so you won't feel a thing or know what's going on during retrieval.

Your eggs are aspirated from your ovaries with a long needle that's inserted through the vaginal wall. Your doctor uses ultrasound to help see where to direct the needle. Sometimes, in addition to aspirating the eggs, your RE will also flush the follicle out with fluid to make sure that she got your egg. If you have fewer than three follicles, your RE will likely aspirate and flush to ensure that she didn't miss the egg.

Afterward, you will wake up in a recovery room. Depending on what medication your doctor uses, you may wake up a few minutes after the procedure has been completed (like five or ten minutes). Expect some additional bloating (I know it was bad enough before you had retrieval; you really didn't want any additional pooching) so wear stretchy, loose fitting pants and slip-on shoes, if possible. (Otherwise, your dear partner will have to tie your shoes for you.) Bending at the waist is going to be difficult for a day or so.

Expect some spotting (I actually bled heavily in the recovery room once) for a day or so. Cramping is normal, too. As you wake up and become more aware of your surroundings, your doctor or a nurse will tell you how many eggs they retrieved. You won't know the overall health of these eggs (how many were mature) or whether they fertilized until the day after retrieval. When you're discharged, your doctor should give you a list of side effects and symptoms to watch out for (these are mostly related to OHSS). If bleeding, bloating, or cramping is excessive, call your doctor's office right away. You will need someone to be with you to drive or escort you home, as you'll be slightly out of it for a while from the anesthesia. Plan to sleep most of the day.

You will begin taking antibiotics and a mild steroid (generally Medrol) to help prevent infection and reduce any inflammation that could interfere with implantation. The next day your doctor's office will call to tell you how many eggs were retrieved, how many were mature, and how many fertilized.

It is possible—God, I hate to say this—that you'll find out that none of your eggs fertilized or that none of them survived after fertilization. This can be devastating and warrants a follow-up call with your doctor. If you do get this awful news, try to remember that not every IVF cycle goes badly, and if you feel strong enough to try again, you may have a completely different outcome. (You can read about what to ask your doctor in chapter 13, on dealing with failed cycles.)

If your eggs fertilized, you will be given a date and time for transfer, depending on whether you're doing a day-3, day-5 or day-6 transfer. (The next section talks about why there are different times to transfer embryos.)

From now until transfer, you will rest and recuperate. You may be bloated, sore, and uncomfortable. You'll also probably obsess about your growing embryos.

This can be a tricky time. You need to be prepared for a call telling you to come in earlier than you were initially told (day 3 instead of day 5), or you may be called and told to come in later (day 5 instead of day 3). This doesn't happen frequently, but it can happen, and it can be very jarring. If it happens, and your transfer date is being moved up (from day 5 to day 3), tell yourself that the safest possible place for your embryos is inside you. If you're being told to wait an extra two days so your embryos can perhaps grow to blastocyst stage (discussed in the next section), remember that your embryologist is trying to give you the best possible chance of getting pregnant while reducing your risk of conceiving triplets. You may freak out about the possibility that your embryos won't survive to day 5 (who wouldn't freak out?). Keep in mind that your embryologist doesn't suggest this unless she thinks you have some good-looking embryos, and it will really help her pick the best possible embryos to transfer. Whenever your transfer is, trust your doctor's and embryologist's judgment. Again, you are paying these folks the big bucks for a reason; this is when they earn it.

## EMBRYO QUALITY, DAY-3, DAY-5, AND DAY-6 BLASTOCYST TRANSFERS, AND ASSISTED HATCHING EXPLAINED

Normal, healthy embryos should cleave (divide) and have two cells about twenty-four to twenty-six hours after fertilization (depending on whether ICSI was used to achieve fertilization). By day 3 (three days after retrieval, retrieval counting as day 0), a normal healthy embryo should have about eight cells. There will be some variation, and not all embryos will be eight cells, but eight is considered ideal. Embryos should be round, with a shell (called the zona pellucida) of uniform thickness all the way around the embryo. The cells within the embryo (called blastomeres) should all be about the same size and shape. Ideally, you want the embryo to be free of small cellular particles, called fragmentation.

Fragmentation looks like a speckled pattern within the embryo, like lots of little tiny cells cluttering up inside the bigger cells, the blastomeres, and the space between the cells and the inner wall of the embryo's shell. The growing embryo will metabolize some fragmentation naturally, but it can also be removed with a vacuum technique performed by the embryologist. Generally, most clinics want to transfer embryos with less than 10 percent fragmentation.

The embryologist grades the embryos based on the number of blastomeres or cells, the overall shape of the embryo and its blastomeres (round or oval), and the amount of fragmentation contained within the embryo. Embryos are generally graded on a scale of 1 to 5, with 1 being the highest and best grade. Every clinic scores embryos slightly differently, attributing more or less points to different characteristics of the embryo and its development.

Embryo grading is *highly subjective*. Two different clinics can give different grades to the same embryo. Whatever grade your embryos receive, it is very important to realize that even poor-quality embryos go on to make healthy babies, and unfortunately some great-quality embryos don't result in a pregnancy. You can never tell what will produce a baby and what won't. Generally speaking, however, transferring three grade 1, eight-celled embryos on day 3 is more likely than not to result in a pregnancy. You can take a look at some pictures of embryos at various stages of growth in the Appendix.

I'm sure you're absolutely dying to know exactly what this day-3 and day-5 transfer is all about. There are three different times to transfer embryos back to your uterus. The first opportunity is three days after retrieval (remember that retrieval counts as day 0). The second occurs five or six days after retrieval. By day 3, healthy embryos will have divided into about eight cells, and by day 5, the healthiest surviving embryos will have divided into two distinct segments or parts; one part or segment will turn into the baby, and the other will turn into the placenta. This segmentation is known as the blastocyst stage of embryo development. Blastocyst transfers are performed on day 5 or day 6 after retrieval. So let's say you have retrieval on a Wednesday. With a day-3 transfer, your embryos will be transferred on Saturday, and with a day-5 transfer, your blastocysts will be transferred on Monday.

Whether they are inside or outside of you, in order to turn into a baby, embryos must develop into blastocysts. Only the healthiest embryos will develop into blastocysts; not all embryos make it to this stage. This is a critical and defining stage of embryo development. An embryo that makes it to "blast" (as it is fondly known) is especially healthy.

It is especially important with IVF, because the culture medium (the solution the embryos are placed in that gives them nourishment to help them grow and develop) doesn't completely match or mimic the nutritional components present in the female reproductive tract. The mediums used today are far superior to those used even two years ago, but even so, there are still problems with quality. The culture mediums can differ from clinic to clinic, and quality can vary even between different batches produced by the same manufacturer. If not all embryos can survive to blast inside you, where the conditions to help them achieve this development are the most ideal, then the conditions to help them grow to this stage outside of your body have to be amazingly perfect. Because culture medium in general isn't as great a source of nutrients for the embryos as that created by your body, and all embryology labs are not alike (some are much better than others), some embryos might make it to blast inside you but not in an embryology lab.

It is critical to have an exceptional embryology lab if you want to have a realistic option of taking your embryos to blast. If there aren't a lot of embryos to work with, it can be risky to take them to blast wherever you are and an even bigger risk at a clinic that doesn't have great success rates for day-3 transfers. If the clinic doesn't get a lot of implantations and pregnancies from day-3 transfers, there probably are issues with the lab or culture medium that will likely preclude your embryos from growing to blast (this is why the lab is so important). You might be able to achieve a pregnancy doing a day-3 transfer with embryos that might arrest (die) while trying to be cultured to blastocyst stage because the conditions outside your body aren't as optimal as those inside you.

The flip side of this day-3/day-5 transfer decision is that the embryos that make it to blast are more likely to result in a pregnancy. Remember that even inside you not all embryos will achieve blastocyst stage, so those that achieve it outside your body are exceptionally hearty. You can transfer fewer of them and still get pregnant while simultaneously reducing the risk of a high-order multiple birth (more than twins). In other words, transferring two blastocysts may have better long-term results than transferring four eight-celled embryos. In good clinics with good labs, blast transfer can have implantation rates as high as 40 percent per embryo, with pregnancy rates over 70 percent per transfer.

In the case of women with high numbers of embryos, doing a day-5 or even a day-6 blastocyst transfer allows the embryos to self-select. One of my very good friends had an embarrassing wealth of embryos (thirteen of them). Her doctors decided to take her to blast, but on day 5, she still had several embryos (six of them). Despite the risk of losing embryos between day 5 and day 6, my friend agreed to go one more day. She lost two more embryos between day 5 and day 6, and two of the remaining four embryos on day 6 were starting to arrest (stop growing). Her doctors were relieved and delighted that they went the extra day. The two blastocysts that were transferred to my friend on day 6 were not the ones they would have chosen on day 5. My friend, by the way, initially conceived twins. Unfortunately, she experienced something called vanishing twin syndrome (it's surprisingly common) and lost one of the pregnancy sacs very early on. She did, however, deliver a beautiful baby girl.

How will your embryologist and doctor make the decision whether to take you to blast? Some clinics almost exclusively perform blast transfers because it lowers the risk of high-order multiple births. Because there is a real risk of losing embryos between day 3 and day 5, some clinics are conservative about culturing to day 5. Some clinics refuse to take the risk at all.

The bottom line is that while blastocyst transfer is much hyped, it remains a very controversial new technology. Many patients think that blast transfers are the goal of an IVF cycle and offer the highest chance of pregnancy. The current thinking, however, is that blast transfer holds a lot of promise, but it's currently best used to reduce the risk of high-order multiple pregnancies. Indeed, some of the clinics and REs that make it a policy *only* to perform blast transfers are demonstrating some of the poorest overall pregnancy rates. When discussing whether you should consider a day-3 or blastocyst transfer, try to remember that this technology will help you balance your goal of achieving pregnancy with the risk that you might wind up with a high-order multiple pregnancy. Talk frankly with your RE and/or embryologist about the number and quality of your embryos before you make assumptions about whether a blastocyst transfer is right for you.

There is one last thing you need to know about embryos. Normally, embryos hatch out of their shell (the zona pellucida) to implant in the embryo wall. Sometimes an embryo will have a thick shell that could impair the ability of the embryo to successfully hatch. The embryologist can pierce the zona pellucida by drilling a small hole through which the embryo can hatch. This is called assisted hatching.

Initially, assisted hatching was heralded as a new technology that increased implantation rates. Current research, however, indicates that assisted hatching does not result in higher implantation rates. Accordingly, most embryologists now feel it appropriate to perform assisted hatching only to remove fragmentation from an embryo or where the zona pellucida is thick or abnormal. The exception is for day-5 or day-6 transfers, in which case your embryologist may routinely perform assisted hatching (some embryologists believe blastocysts need a little extra help to hatch).

Because assisted hatching is usually done selectively (based on each embryo's need for it), it's possible to transfer four embryos on day 3 and have one or two of them, but not all, receive assisted hatching. I have had assisted hatching performed on my embryos and thought that this was a sign that the embryo wasn't healthy. Because I got pregnant from that group of embryos—and have no way of knowing which embryo implanted, the ones with the assisted hatching or the ones without—I don't know that this was necessarily the right conclusion. Assisted hatching may have helped me get pregnant that cycle. Who knows? If you have assisted hatching, think of it as extra insurance.

## IVF PATIENTS AND EMBRYO TRANSFER

The transfer procedure can be performed a couple of different ways. However it's accomplished, you want it to be untraumatic for your embryos. Embryos are extremely fragile and can easily be damaged during transfer, thereby reducing your chance of getting pregnant. In fact, from a medical standpoint, almost everything that has occurred in your IVF cycle is meaningless if you have a bad transfer; this is the most critical part of your cycle. It is so important that some clinics grade transfer (in addition to embryo quality) to determine how likely you are to get pregnant. Embryo grading and transfer grading are used for research purposes to help your doctor or clinic determine the best situations for achieving pregnancies.

To accomplish an easy transfer, some clinics rely on ultrasound. After you drink a gallon of water so you have a full bladder (ugh!) to help your doctor see what she is doing, she will perform an ultrasound to help position the catheter in your uterus through which the embryos will be inserted. Other clinics (like mine) perform a mock transfer before your IVF cycle starts and map where the catheter needs to be placed, noting curves and bends and various measurements along the way. Both techniques help your doctor perform an easy transfer, but from what I hear, the ultrasound-guided transfer can be pretty uncomfortable because of the full bladder and tender postretrieval ovaries.

Transfer itself (the catheter insertion and placement) should be relatively painless. Sometimes the catheter hurts a little bit as it inserted through your cervix, and sometimes there's some cramping from its presence in your uterus. Some centers have big television screens that have a picture of your embryos for you to look at during the procedure. And you will probably be given an opportunity to talk to the embryologist about your embryos. You may even be given a photograph of the embryos and a report card (telling you the cell stage of each embryo) to take home with you. I have included pictures of some embryos in the Appendix.

After transfer, you'll go to a recovery area where you can rest. Some clinics ask you to lie in a specific position, while others just want you to be still for a few minutes. Report any uncomfortable cramping either during or immediately after the procedure and any cramping that occurs continuously for more than twenty-four hours after your transfer. After discharge, stay quiet for a few days. Some clinics ask you to stay on strict bed rest for at least forty-eight hours; others ask only that you rest and watch a lot of television or read in bed for a couple of days. Try to avoid going back to work for two days or so.

You are now officially in the two-week wait, the hell that precedes your pregnancy test! Now, a lot of people wonder whether they should just plunk themselves down in bed for the entire two weeks before their pregnancy test. You can if you want to, if you have the resources to do it. I read on the Internet about a woman who rented a hospital bed and made her husband empty bed pans. She literally never got out of bed, except maybe to shower, I hope. This is definitely *not* necessary! Think about women who don't go through infertility treatment. They go out and live their lives without giving a thought to what's going on inside them. If they can achieve implantation this way, then so can you. Just don't smoke, drink excessively, or use drugs or certain medications (over-the-counter or otherwise).

Don't go for a two-mile run right now or engage in any kind of vigorous exercise or heavy (more than ten pounds) lifting. *Caution* is the word of posttransfer life. You've just paid a ton of money and gone through a physically demanding series of injections and procedures. Why jeopardize your outcome for a workout? Follow all doctor's instructions (like no sex or orgasms until after your pregnancy test), take it easy, and get lots of sleep and eat well. If you have a question about what you can and can't do, call your doctor or IVF nurse.

A lot of people worry that laughing or coughing after transfer, or even straining for a bowel movement will dislodge or cause the embryos to be expelled. That's not going to happen! (And let's face it; the progesterone is going to make you constipated, so you're going to be straining at some point!) If you start bleeding heavily after transfer and start passing tissue (like you would with a period) call your doctor. But being consti-pated or having bronchitis isn't something to worry about (except from a discomfort standpoint).

## FROZEN EMBRYO TRANSFERS (FET)

Sometimes you'll leave transfer knowing that your extra embryos are be-ing frozen; other times you are told the other embryos will be observed for a few days before a determination will be made as to whether to freeze them. When do embryos get frozen, and why do they get frozen?

Well, if you are lucky enough to have so many healthy embryos they can't all be transferred to your uterus at one time, you don't want to just throw out the extras. Mercifully, medical science developed a way to freeze and then thaw embryos you don't use right away, so you can use them if you miscarry, fail to get pregnant from your initial transfer of fresh embryos (nonfrozen embryos), or want to create a sibling for the baby you did conceive after the initial fresh transfer. This sibling would actually be a fraternal twin to your older child, even though they don't gestate at the same time. Deciding when to freeze embryos is a little more complicated.

Some clinics freeze everything that is left over on day 3. Other centers wait until day 5 and freeze only what has made it to blast. If the option of a frozen transfer is important to you, make it your business to find out *before* you cycle what your doctor's criteria are for freezing embryos. The one and only thing I regret about where I cycled is that they didn't do as many frozen transfers as some clinics. If I had it to do again, I might have tried one cycle at a clinic that was more likely to freeze my extra embryos (even those that didn't seem "perfect"). I have one very good friend who has the most wonderful little boy from an FET. From what Lori has described to me about the quality of the embryos she had frozen, I know that my clinic would never have frozen his embryo. I still wonder in the middle of the night whether certain of my discarded embryos might have been frozen had I been at a more liberal fertility clinic. It's not a nice thought; avoid it if you can.

FETs tend to be more successful if you got pregnant from the fresh (nonfrozen) embryos transferred from the same cycle (same batch). If you got pregnant from the fresh batch, the entire batch of embryos created at that time (which includes those you had frozen) is considered "pregnancy worthy." If you didn't get pregnant from the fresh transfer, you still can get pregnant from the frozen embryos, but statistically it's less likely.

FETs aren't as successful as fresh IVF transfers. How successful FETs are depends on where you are. Some clinics have better protocols and facilities for freezing and thawing embryos that give you better chances of having healthy frozen embryos with which to get pregnant. Some perform many more FETs and have higher success rates because they do it all the time, and they know how to do it well. But plenty of women get pregnant from FETs performed at smaller centers.

On average, an FET that is managed with medications to prepare the uterus for implantation, known as a "program FET" (we'll talk more about what this means in one second), with three healthy thawed embryos will give you about a 35 percent chance of conceiving. The statistics are slightly lower for natural-cycle FETs that rely on your natural menstrual cycle to prepare the body for implantation, and when you're transferring a smaller number of embryos. Your chances are probably better than that of the average twenty-five-year-old trying to conceive, but not as high as they can be with a fresh IVF transfer.

Deciding whether to do a natural or program FET may be out of your control; some clinics will only do program FETs. If you have the choice, you should consider which option is better for you. (Some women welcome a cycle without needles, even though it has a lower chance of succeeding.)

In a natural FET cycle, your RE monitors your body for ovulation by following you with ultrasounds and blood work. When you have achieved a healthy ovulation, your doctor will schedule your embryo transfer. If you do not evidence a healthy ovulation, your doctor may ask you to try again another month rather than risk transferring embryos into an environment that isn't quite healthy enough to receive and support them. Your embryos will be thawed and then transferred back to your uterus, and you will wait to see if you get pregnant. This is an easy way to do FET, and it is successful (it was for Lori). Many women—and some doctors—feel this is more successful than the program FET (that I will discuss in a moment), because your body is free of chemicals and hormones that might adversely affect implantation and pregnancy development. There is even research done to see if freezing embryos soon after fertilization and then transferring them in a cycle where the mother is hormone free and does not need luteal support (like progesterone injections or estrogen pills) can result in higher pregnancy rates. Statistically, however, program FETs are more successful.

Program FETs are performed with chemical support to ensure a proper uterine environment to maximize the likelihood of achieving implantation and pregnancy. With a program FET, your menstrual cycle is suppressed (usually with Lupron). You take estrogen (generally patches that stick to your belly, but you might also take injections or pills) to build up your uterine lining. Every couple of days your estrogen dosage increases, which further stimulates the development of the lining. The growth of your lining is monitored by ultrasound. Your E2 level will be monitored by blood work. You continue to take Lupron throughout this time.

At about CD15 of your FET cycle, your estrogen dose is decreased, and you begin taking tetracycline or another antibiotic, and Medrol just as you would after retrieval with a fresh (as in not frozen) cycle. You will also begin progesterone support (generally through IM injection). On or about CD17, you will go in for transfer of your embryos. Afterward, you will continue the estrogen and progesterone support and follow usual posttransfer protocols. If you are doing a frozen blast transfer, the protocol I outlined may differ somewhat from yours. Specifically, your transfer will occur later in the cycle than for women transferring embryos frozen on or before day-3.

When you go for transfer, you need to be prepared for a couple of things. First, not all of your embryos may have thawed successfully. Success with thawing varies from clinic to clinic (again, another reason to be at a state-of-the-art facility with a great embryology lab), but even with the best that science and medicine has to offer, some embryos don't survive. It is also not uncommon to have embryos lose cells (blastomeres) when thawing. In the best of all possible worlds—and this is a gumption trap; don't expect this to happen or you might be horribly disappointed when it doesn't—all of your embryos survive, thaw, and grow before transfer. You can, however, get pregnant from embryos that lose cells or don't grow after they are thawed. Don't freak out if your embryos aren't perfect after thawing; they usually aren't.

## THE DREADED TWO-WEEK WAIT

Welcome to what I think is the worst part of infertility treatment. There's not much you can do during the dreaded two weeks when you wait to find out if you're pregnant, so mostly you'll just rest and obsess. You will overanalyze every twinge, cramp, and gas bubble. Let me tell you something that Dr. Chung told me: "Early pregnancy symptoms are notoriously unreliable." I have been pregnant and had no symptoms, and I've been pregnant and been sick as a dog from about one week after transfer. There's no real way to tell whether you are pregnant or not without that blood test.

What are some of the symptoms you might be feeling, and what might be something to worry about? Well, spotting and cramping after transfer is completely normal. If this doesn't stop in a day or two, call your doctor. Bleeding is not normal, so be careful to distinguish bleeding from spotting. You should not need a maxipad. A panty liner should be enough. Anything more than that, and you should give a call to your doctor to make sure it's okay. Cramping that doesn't subside within a day or so also warrants a call.

Implantation spotting is another thing you surely will be looking for. Many women report having some spotting or bleeding several days after transfer during cycles in which they got pregnant. This can occur a few days after transfer or right around the time when your period is due. Most people think implantation should be finished by this time, but the process lasts for a couple of weeks, and the most intense period when embryos make their strongest attachment to the uterine wall may occur just before or around when your period is due. I can't tell you how many women I have known who have assumed that the spotting they experienced was the beginning of their period, and were devastated. They wanted to stop taking their progesterone support. Had they stopped, they might have seriously jeopardized what turned out to be healthy pregnancies. If you have any questions about spotting, call your doctor. Be cautious, follow your doctor's instructions, and try not to overthink it.

Another big subject for obsession during the two-week wait is: when should implantation after IVF take place? Doctors aren't really sure. After a day-3 transfer, implantation is most likely to take place during the next forty-eight to seventy-two hours. After a day-5 or day-6 transfer, implantation should take place during the next twenty-four to forty-eight hours. With an IUI, implantation should take place about five days after insemination. But that doesn't mean that every embryo implants during this window of time.

Everyone thinks that sore breasts are another sign of pregnancy. I have news for you on this one. I think this is a crock! Ninety percent of my friends and I never had boob issues until well into our pregnancies. Don't, I repeat, *don't* expect your breasts to tell you whether you might be pregnant.

You might experience mood swings during the two-week wait. It is probably a combination of stress and hormones making you insane now— and by the way, when I say insane, I mean totally *off-the-wall crazy*. This is the most emotionally demanding time of IUI/IVF, waiting and won-

**A word to the wise:** | If you are taking progesterone, especially progesterone in oil, you should not expect to get your period while taking the medicine. Although some women do get their period on progesterone, most women don't. The progesterone should suppress your menstrual bleeding. If you are bleeding while you are taking progesterone in oil (or another form of it), you should call your doctor.

dering if you are pregnant. The fear of not being pregnant is enough to induce most of us to commit ourselves to the nearest psychiatric facility.

## YOUR PREGNANCY TEST

The big day is drawing near, and you must be as nervous as you've ever been. Did the cycle work? Am I pregnant? Am I carrying multiples? Why don't my boobs hurt (or, if you're like me, wondering if they hurt from all the pinching and poking you're doing or because you're pregnant)?

I had so many bad experiences with negative results when Charlie and I were doing inseminations. I *hated* the day of the big phone call with the results. Then the first time I did IVF—and had the best chances of conceiving and the highest hopes I'd had up to that point—the cycle failed. It was beyond devastating. I don't think I ever cried so much in my life. Between the negative IUI pregnancy tests and that negative IVF pregnancy test, I really and truly think I developed a form of post-traumatic stress disorder (I call it post-traumatic stress infertility disorder). The big phone call became a nightmare experience for me.

If you find waiting for the phone call is stressful, think of creative ways to reduce your anxiety. Have your doctor's office call your husband or partner. Let your answering machine take the message. Have the clinic call your cell phone and then turn it off and hide it in a drawer until you and your partner can listen to the message together. If this day gets unduly stressful, you do have the power to make it easier on yourself. Now let's talk about the results and what they mean.

# 13

# Finding Out If Your Cycle Was Successful

After all the needles, drugs, multiple procedures, and obsession about egg or embryo quality, you're ready to have the all-important beta HCG blood test (the beta). You're about as calm as a woman who lost her child in a department store!

You may be thrilled, devastated, or even confused by your beta results. This chapter will explain all about home pregnancy tests and beta results and what they mean (it's not always as straightforward as we'd like), talk about what it's like to be pregnant finally (surprisingly, sometimes it's not always as joyful as we want it to be), and discuss what to do if—God forbid—you're not pregnant (aside from wanting to crawl into bed for the next ten years).

## All About Betas and Home Pregnancy Tests

You've probably been wrestling with your desire to take a home pregnancy test (HPT) before beta day arrives. HPTs are evil. *Evil,* I tell you!

Did you know that you could get a negative HPT the day of your beta and go in and have your blood test and learn that you are in fact pregnant? While HPT manufacturers claim 99 percent accuracy, in the world of infertility, HPTs are about as reliable as most babysitters. The only women I've ever known (or heard about) who got a reliable positive HPT before their beta were women expecting multiples. Most of us get negative HPT results even when we're pregnant!

If you ignore my advice and take an HPT before beta day, there are two things you need to know. First, do *not* take your HPT until at least *ten days past your transfer or twelve days past insemination.* This ensures that you've (probably) completely metabolized the HCG from your trigger injection and any positive result you get is more likely than not to be accurate. Second, if the test is negative *do not*—I repeat—*do not* freak out and *assume you're not pregnant.* Many, many women will get a negative HPT, even when they have a healthy, positive result from their beta HCG blood test. Studies have been done that show HPTs regularly miss early IUI and IVF pregnancies. Your beta is about a thousand times more reliable than your HPT. So do yourself a favor; if you pee on that stick, take your HPT results with a *huge* grain of salt.

Beta HCG blood tests can detect HCG in your system in minute quantities. A beta will be considered positive with any quantitative value greater than 5. Most HPTs are standardized and will test positive only when you've got roughly the amount of HCG that most women have in their system *two days after* they've missed their period—or two days after when your first beta is taken. This corresponds roughly to a beta result of 100. Yet many healthy initial (first) betas come back well under 100. So you tell me, why take an HPT and risk getting a negative result when your beta is so much more sensitive and might be positive despite the negative HPT (and you avoid the stress that comes with a negative HPT)? And even more important to consider is that HCG levels can vary significantly among women.

Some women with healthy viable pregnancies have very low HCG levels at first and others have extremely high levels (even with singleton pregnancies). Your beta HCG level will tell you exactly the amount of

HCG in your system. You'll know if you're pregnant even if you have a beta as low as ten. This is why I refused to take HPTs. I knew that my beta would tell me conclusively whether I was pregnant; I don't like being tortured with inconclusive pregnancy test results. Now that's not to say that beta HCG blood work is always as definitive as I like things to be. In my book, a positive result is a positive! Not so for my RE.

There are certain levels of HCG that REs like to see from your initial beta. Most clinics like to see an initial beta of 50 approximately eleven days past a day-3 transfer, or fourteen days past an IUI or retrieval/fertilization. And they like to see the level double every forty-eight to seventy-two hours. Every clinic has its own standards for what a healthy beta is and at what intervals betas need to be repeated. (Yes, you're going to have go through the waiting again!) If your beta is above the level your clinic or RE deems acceptable, you get a wonderful phone call with your results! *Yippee!* If your initial beta fails to fulfill your clinic's expectations of a healthy result, you get a less-than-reassuring congratulatory call from your clinic. My least favorite response was: "Well, Liz, your beta was positive, *but* it's a little low, and we're somewhat concerned." That's not good news to anyone's ears, especially someone who's been obsessing and worrying for two weeks!

If your beta is a little low in the beginning, it doesn't mean your pregnancy isn't viable. It only means your pregnancy needs to be closely monitored. The lower the number, the more cause there is for concern. If you have a low initial beta, most clinics ask that you repeat the blood work again in forty-eight hours. Your clinic will be looking to see if your beta doubled in that time frame (it should double every forty-eight to seventy-two hours). If it just barely doubled, you may need to come in again for more blood work (this varies from clinic to clinic). Sometimes, however, when you repeat the blood work, your beta will drop. This is generally an indication that the pregnancy is ending. Of course, your first beta might come back at a very healthy 150, in which case you might not need to repeat the blood work at all, or more likely repeat it a week later. It's up to your clinic whether they'll want you to repeat your beta when it comes back with a healthy initial result.

The other thing that "but" can mean when you get your pregnancy test results is that you're carrying multiples! To your doctor, a very high beta can be a cause for concern just as a low beta can be. My friend Diane had an initial beta of 900; she was carrying triplets. Now, while you may be rejoicing at the thought of having multiples, most fertility centers consider a high-order multiple pregnancy (triplets or more) to be a management failure. What is a blessing to you is a potential medical nightmare to them.

Fertility doctors are constantly seeking new ways to reduce the risk of high-order multiple pregnancy requiring selective reduction. Selective reduction is a process by which the pregnancy is reduced from quadruplets or triplets to twins or even a singleton. Having to decide whether to do selective reduction is *gut wrenching*. The procedure itself is risky; choosing to forgo it can jeopardize the pregnancy for both mother and babies. Selective reduction is a very personal decision. No one should judge what a couple decides to do when faced with a high-order multiple pregnancy. Multiple pregnancies aren't easy (and just think of all those diapers!), but they can turn out just fine.

But don't focus too much on this stuff. This is another time to let your RE sweat it out while you try to relax (easier said than done, I know). It is also important to realize that some clinics have a much more relaxed attitude and others are hypervigilant. Take your blood test results with a grain of salt.

Once you hit higher numbers—around 2,000 give or take—your beta may stop doubling every forty-eight hours. It still will continue to rise slowly until it plateaus toward the end of your first trimester. Your HCG level will then gradually drop off. The normal ranges for HCG levels (singleton and/or multiple pregnancies) look something like this. Note that there is quite a large range for "normal." (I also gave you a link to HCG levels broken down by day and by singleton/multiple pregnancy in the Resources section.)

| Weeks of Pregnancy | Serum HCG level |
|---|---|
| 3–4 | 9–130 |
| 4–5 | 75–2,600 |
| 5–6 | 850–20,800 |
| 6–7 | 4,000–100,200 |
| 7–12 | 11,500–289,000 |
| 12–16 | 18,300–137,000 |
| 16–29 (2nd trimester) | 1,400–53,000 |
| 29–41 (3rd trimester) | 1,400–60,000 |

Betas are funny things. You really need to be Zen about them because they can do just about anything (including drive you over the edge). My friend Sarah's initial beta came back at 12. Her betas were repeated every forty-eight hours for almost three weeks and were still low and barely doubling between tests. Even after Sarah saw a heartbeat on her ultrasound (normally the all-clear sign) her RE told her not to get her hopes up; her beta was still so low that he couldn't imagine that this was a viable pregnancy. Sarah was a wreck for weeks. Her daughter was born nine months later. Statistically, Sarah's pregnancy shouldn't have carried to term, but it did. All the stress she endured worrying about the betas spoiled the joy of her pregnancy.

Whatever your initial positive result may be, take a deep breath! If it's negative, have faith; the odds are in your favor that you will get pregnant and go on to have a healthy baby. In the meantime, skip ahead and read about what to do when you get bad news. If you got good news, well a positive—however low or high it may be—is a *positive,* and that means you're *pregnant!* Let your doctor worry about whether the numbers are where they should be and are doubling properly.

## You're Pregnant!

Once you get over the initial shock (and bliss!), you might be a little surprised at your reaction to news of your pregnancy. Most women who get pregnant after infertility treatment are terrified something will go wrong. And the fear doesn't go away.

If you let the fear rule the process of having blood tests, how are you going to react when your early ultrasounds have to be repeated (most women have at least two ultrasounds before being discharged to an OB-GYN) or deal with the *normal* stress and fear associated with a developing pregnancy? And if you start to depend too much on blood work and ultrasounds to tell you that everything is "normal" and "fine," you're setting a bad precedent for the next nine months.

After going in for daily blood work and ultrasounds during your cycle and then having repeat blood work and ultrasounds during early pregnancy, it's a huge shock to suddenly go a month without seeing a doctor. If you need extra reassurance from your doctor that things are progressing normally, ask your OB to schedule an extra ultrasound. Talk frankly with her about your fears and concerns and ask for extra support. You worked hard for this pregnancy; it's okay to feel fragile and afraid.

The second shocker is that not all of your cycle buddies are going to be happy for you. This leaves most of us with an odd mix of anger and guilt. If you ask me, you have every right to be angry. While I'll admit to being a little jealous at first, I also was always happy for my friends who got pregnant from treatment. It reminded me that it works! The guilt is tougher to deal with.

Survivor's guilt—the guilt you experience for surviving and moving past your infertility when others haven't—cannot rule your life. It's normal to have some guilt in the beginning, and it's normal to have some trouble communicating with people still enduring infertility. Listening to them as they continue to wrestle with the ups and downs may be more than you can handle. But please try not to feel guilty that your cycle worked. Today is *your* day.

So how are you going to celebrate? Are you going to go buy baby furniture or tell your friends or family? Many people will caution you against making announcements or purchases until you're at least in your second trimester, but I don't know that I agree with this approach. I believe in *celebrating* pregnancy!

If celebrating means telling your friends and family, I think you should go for it. If something unspeakable happens later on down the road, you'll have more support as you manage your grief. It may not be a good idea to tell the whole world right away. Consider the chart you made in chapter 8, and anyone who you would want to know that you miscarried should be someone you tell about your pregnancy. If you want to go buy cute little baby clothes and wash them and put them in the new changing table you ordered, *do it* (just make sure to wash the clothes in Dreft or Ivory Snow)!

## Negative Betas, Failed Cycles, and Miscarriage

If your beta wasn't positive, I'm so, so sorry! My very first IVF cycle was a dismal failure, and I was devastated for weeks. It's really kind of like having a miscarriage. And if you did IVF, well, you know there were embryos—babies—inside you. I know a lot of REs don't like to call them embryos and instead call them preembryos. They don't want you to start thinking about them as little life forms, as babies. But you know in your heart that those are your babies.

The failure of an IUI or IVF cycle is much more difficult to bear than the failure of a cycle trying to make a baby the old-fashioned way. So much more effort goes into it! Needles and mood swings, physical discomfort, blood tests, ultrasounds, procedure after procedure; it's a lot. I remember Dr. Chung telling me that for every six phone calls he made congratulating couples, he had to make four phone calls consoling families over the cycle's failure. I hated being one of those four couples. I hated losing, I hated failing, I hated not being pregnant, *again!*

If your cycle resulted in a negative beta, make an appointment and talk face-to-face with your RE (no phone sessions, go *see* her and get her undivided attention). Get a sense of what your RE thinks of your E2 level, follicle development, semen analysis (if you did IUI), your egg and embryo quality (if you did IVF). If it was your first IVF cycle, it's even more imperative that you talk with your RE. This is where the diagnostic component of IVF comes into play. Your RE has now seen you through a cycle and learned a lot about your egg and embryos and response to various drugs. Now she can really work on improving and fixing things she didn't even know were going wrong. If it wasn't your first cycle, find out if she thinks there are things you can do to improve the chances of achieving a pregnancy next time. Discuss embryo coculture programs, different combinations of drugs, and a slower or faster stims phase. What about using donor material or a surrogate? You always have options! Make sure you talk with your RE in detail about what choices you have if you want to continue treatment.

Even more devastating than a negative beta comes when you learn that your pregnancy isn't viable. Though low initial betas or dropping betas are an indication you might want to prepare yourself for miscarriage, often no warning comes. The good news—if there is any—is that women who conceive with IVF and then miscarry are more likely to conceive and carry to term than women who fail to get pregnant with IVF. Small consolation, I know.

If your pregnancy is more than six weeks along when you find out about your loss, talk with your RE about having a D & C to obtain pregnancy tissue for a pathologist's analysis. Many women prefer to bleed and miscarry on their own, but if you choose this route, there is no way to find out what caused the miscarriage. The pathology and genetic reports obtained from the D & C can provide information that will help your RE guide your treatment. You might learn that you could benefit from a complete genetic (karyotype) workup, a visit with a genetic counselor, or trying PGD (see chapter 7).

I had D & Cs for two of my miscarriages. Each time I got results from the hospital indicating that I was carrying a normal healthy baby girl. When you find out you were carrying a baby girl, there is always the chance that the tissue that was sampled was your tissue and not that of the embryo. It is only when the pathology indicates you were carrying a girl with a chromosomal error (since you're alive, science will presume you don't have any problems with your chromosomes) or were carrying a boy (either normal chromosomes or not, the tissue sampled could not have been yours because you don't carry the Y chromosome) that you can be absolutely certain that the tissue sampled was the baby's. But the likelihood that you'll get ambiguous results is far outweighed by the possibility that you'll learn something helpful.

Even if you don't get any substantively helpful information, I think a D & C is far easier than suffering through a miscarriage on your own. Not only is it less painful (the D & C is a fairly easy surgical procedure with minimal postoperative bleeding and cramping) but it's also much less messy. Passing fetal tissue naturally can be acutely painful. Your bleeding is heavier, clottier, and clumpier than normal. I've miscarried both ways, and let me tell you, I'd much rather face the IV needle and an operating room (oh my God, did I really just say that?) than bleed that pregnancy tissue out on my own. Besides, who wants to run the risk that you won't pass all the tissue and wind up having to have a D & C anyway, and taking antibiotics to avoid infection? Trust me on this one. If your pregnancy has progressed far enough along (usually more than six weeks) to indicate that a D & C might be appropriate, *do it!*

If you suffer a miscarriage after treatment, take time to grieve and heal. Don't rush back into treatment. You need to let your hormone levels return to normal and give your body time to heal. Depending on how far along in your pregnancy you were, this can take a while. Some doctors may want you to wait three months before cycling again. You also need time to let go of the dreams and hopes that came with that pregnancy. Rushing back into treatment and getting pregnant again right away will not make the pain go away. Another pregnancy cannot replace the baby you just lost or lessen your grief. Find a support group for pregnancy loss or a counselor or therapist, write in a journal, or scream into your pillow. It's okay to acknowledge that you feel like a part of you just died (it did) and that you're angry that this is so hard (it is really hard, *infuriatingly* hard)! Once you come face-to-face with the pain and anger, it will begin to dissipate. I'm still working through grief more than a year after my last miscarriage, because I didn't take the time to move through my sadness and pain.

Even if you haven't suffered a miscarriage, taking some downtime in between cycles is incredibly important. You need to recharge your batteries, because you need them to function at full strength if you're going to get through another cycle. But more importantly—and this is my completely medically undocumented, personal opinion—I really think giving your body a break from the hormones helps you respond better to the drugs the next time you cycle. I always had fewer side effects and a better response to the drugs when I had taken a couple of months off between treatment cycles.

Now I know you don't want to take a break. You probably want to jump right back in and try again this instant! The suckiest thing about being infertile and doing IVF is that at most we get a whopping four attempts a year to get pregnant. Compared with the average ten (if not twelve) attempts fertile couples get, you feel pressured to cycle as soon as possible. You want as many chances to conceive as possible, and you want those opportunities to come as soon as possible. Despite the overwhelming need to fill the void and try again, consider taking a break. Get rid of the bad energy from the last cycle; you'll feel better in the long run.

When it's time to face another cycle—whether you've suffered a devastating cycle failure or miscarried at five or ten weeks—it's going to be weird. There's no easy way to do another cycle after you've had a failure or loss. In some respects it seems less daunting because you know what you're facing. But at the same time, it's more frightening because you know more about the things that can go wrong, you know how demanding treatment is, and you know what's at stake. The only way I was ever able to do it was to just *do it*. I didn't think about it; I didn't analyze it, I didn't obsess about it (a first for me!). I just did it. I stocked up on stuff for my care package and distracted myself as much as possible. I went over the Clean Slate Rule with Charlie and made a list of all the things we had learned from the last cycle and all the reasons this cycle was starting with a clean slate.

And then I got up on the morning of my first Lupron injection and went about my day. I set aside something special (a good movie and a nice fattening meal of macaroni and cheese for dinner) for that night to reward me for getting through my first injection of the cycle, and that was it. I was back in the swing of it, and I was okay.

Or maybe you don't want to try again. Maybe it's time to stop and take a break or move forward with your contingency plan. Go back and read about your different options for treatment, the Clean Slate Rule, and making game and contingency plans; perhaps it's time to revise your road map.

Remember you own this experience! You can get off this blasted roller coaster or decide to go for another ride. Put yourself first, and do what's right for *you*.

# 14

# Deciding When It's Time to Move On

ENOUGH, ALREADY!

When you start thinking about stopping treatment, you're pretty much emotionally, physically, and spiritually exhausted. It's a sad and hard time. I faced it many, many times and never examined the issues without crying, often hysterically, for long periods of time. Or perhaps you and your husband agreed when you started treatment that you could only afford one cycle or would only try once. But you still somehow feel it's wrong to stop trying. There are many ways to build a family, and you can have a beautiful, fulfilling life without children as well (I talk about this in chapter 7). But letting go of infertility treatment when you aren't sure you're ready or you have the what-if-next-time-is-the-one syndrome, or you aren't given a choice and your doctor says it's time to move on, what can I say? It's *brutal!*

Stopping IVF was the most difficult decision of my life. Infertility treatment is *addictive*.

That's right. Infertility treatment is addictive, and it's just as hard to stop and move on with your life as it is to give up heroin. I kid you not (and no, I've never been faced with giving up heroin, so I don't really know if it's *exactly* the same, but I have enough friends who are recovering alcoholics or addicts working a twelve step program to know that there are a lot of serious parallels). So maybe you don't get high from injecting yourself with HCG, but believe me the rush of hope that you get with each injection of stims isn't far off. It's a never ending daily, weekly, monthly addiction to the overwhelming rush of maternal hormones and dreams that comes with each injection, each phone call, each procedure, and each pregnancy test. It's almost impossible to give it up. I mean, *think* about it for a moment.

Exactly how incredible is it that you and your partner can spend tens of thousands of dollars and stab yourself with needles of all disgusting sizes? What is it that motivates you to do this? It's that smell of your new baby's fuzzy little head; it's the dream of feeling a baby move inside you, of breast-feeding, of leaving the hospital in a wheelchair carrying a tiny pink or blue bundle, of *your* baby shower and *your* baby announcement! Those are some powerful fantasies you've got going there, especially if they get you through the shots and financial ruin. You want to tell me that the pure, unadulterated rush that comes with those visions of bliss is any less powerful or addictive than narcotic-induced highs?

I'm not saying this to disparage you. You're an incredibly powerful kick-ass kind of woman if you've tried even one cycle using assisted reproductive technologies. The point is that when you feel out of control and overwhelmed, you *are!* There were many times when I felt consumed by my desire to have a child and the tremendous hope of having a child that is created by IVF. Look, reproductive technology offers perpetual hope of having a child. It's almost *impossible* to walk away from that. But sometimes it's necessary.

After four miscarriages, five and half IVF cycles, one FET, four IUIs, two laparoscopies, two hysteroscopies, two D & Cs, and countless injections, I couldn't do it anymore. There was too much grief in my heart to continue. Having a baby isn't about grieving; it's supposed to be a joyous event, and there just wasn't any joy in my life at all.

Even after Charlie and I made the decision to stop medical treatment, I wasn't certain I was doing the right thing. I had to learn to live my life in a new way: without treatments, without cycles to look forward to, without that almost-attainable dream that the next cycle would work and I would carry to term.

Eventually I started to see everything that I had lost during my foray into infertility treatment hell and to enjoy being unencumbered by fantasies, illusions, and visions of what I thought treatment offered me. I could be a mom and breast-feed without being pregnant; what would that be like? I didn't have to live in fear that I would have another miscarriage. I could finally lose all the IVF and pregnancy weight and have my body back! There was a new world in front of me, and gradually I began to explore it and *enjoy* it.

I still have longings for days gone by. I think I probably always will. But mostly it's nice to hear the phone ring and not worry that Dr. Chung's calling me to give me some test results or talk about my next cycle.

So how will you know when it's time to move on? For me, the thought of risking another miscarriage was too scary. I couldn't face another loss and emotionally survive. My heart told me it was time to stop. I just *knew*.

Another way to tell when you are done is when you start to resent everything you're giving up for IVF. When was the last time you went on vacation or could even think about planning a vacation that didn't interfere with your treatment calendar? How about when your bank balance is getting frighteningly low, and you just don't feel comfortable maxing out your fourth credit card, taking out a home equity loan, or refinancing your house for the third time. When you start resenting the cost of treatment and how rich your doctor is getting—and I'm not talking about feeling sarcastic or cynical here, I'm talking about anger—then maybe it's time to reconsider your options.

Deciding to stop when treatment isn't working for you is more difficult. When you've done several cycles of IVF and aren't getting pregnant and you aren't getting answers about why, it may be time to look at your road map or contingency plan and rethink your choices. If you haven't been to a world-renowned fertility clinic, call one. Get a second (or third) opinion, and see what that doctor says. Does he think it's worth trying again?

The hardest situation, however, is when you want to continue treatment but your doctor says she won't treat you anymore. You feel completely abandoned and hopeless. There's always the option of trying another clinic, but if you've already gone to a couple of different places, and/or cycled more than half a dozen times, it's probably wise to consider why your doctor feels that it's a good idea to stop. Sit down and ask her to explain her recommendation.

The trouble with following your doctor's advice and moving on before you feel ready is twofold. First, you've got to contend with the ever-powerful addiction and the fear that you might be giving up the cycle that works (what if next time is the one that works?). Second, you have to deal with the IVF urban legend: the woman who conceived against all odds after an unbelievable twelve cycles of IVF.

We've all heard stories about women like this. I believe they're a myth and only serve to give us false hope. Maybe some woman out there conceived after twelve IVF cycles, but most conscientious and/or respectable doctors won't let women cycle that many times.

Before you strive to become your clinic's urban legend, *think* about it. Do you really want to cycle that many times? Is a biological child that important to you? The genetic link is powerful. But would you have a better chance of conceiving if you used donor eggs or a surrogate? You can breast-feed (is there anything more maternal than *that?*) when you use a surrogate and when you adopt (check out the Resources section for more information). What about adoption? Adoption is a joyous experience, it's guaranteed (that's right, *guaranteed*), and there are no needles involved. Is this something you might consider? What is driving you so hard to have a child that you're willing to try to be that nameless woman who got pregnant on her twelfth IVF cycle?

I have several friends who have tried and tried and tried and never gotten pregnant with IVF. Watching them wrestle with the question of when to let go or what to do when their doctor told them to stop was devastating for me; it must have been a thousand times more devastating for them. By the way, Dr. Chung did tell me after my last miscarriage that he wouldn't let me try IVF again, unless I was planning to use a gestational carrier (an IVF surrogacy). I already knew I was done, but hearing him say it was still unbelievably painful and depressing. If you have chosen your doctors carefully and tried several times, if none of the therapies and treatments you're trying is working, then listening to your doctor and taking a break may be appropriate; devastating, but appropriate. It's easier when your heart tells you it's time to move on; it's nearly impossible when someone else is telling you to stop.

What if you and your partner are at odds? He wants to stop, and you don't. You want to stop, and he doesn't. Either way, there's tension and anger and resentment. A conversation about the local news easily dissolves into a fight over continuing treatment. I've been there, and this is very hard. One thing to consider, however, is that the problems you're facing aren't so much about infertility treatment as they are about communication and trust. (Hey, listen, after four years of marriage counseling, I think I've earned the right to psychoanalyze your marriage!)

Even if you could resolve the infertility issues, there would probably be tension when you have that beautiful baby. I have learned from parenting that babies exacerbate every weakness in a marriage and seriously test even the best marriages. If issues are arising during infertility treatment, deal with them before you move on to parenthood or divorce court.

Whether you're thinking about terminating treatment because of your finances, marital stress, repeated failed cycles, or because you just plain feel like it is time to move on, I applaud you! Whether you choose to live without children, use donor material, use a surrogate, or adopt a beautiful baby or child, you're charting your own path for the first time in a very long time.

There is no one in the world but those of us who have walked away who know the pain this causes you and understand and accept the jealousy and anger in your heart that ART failed you. There is no one in the world but those of us who walked away who know how strong you are, how brave you are, and how scared you are. I salute your integrity, bravery, honesty, and endurance!

# 15

# Making Your Infertility Work for You

### YES, INFERTILITY CAN BE A GOOD THING

Last night at three o'clock in the morning, I held my whimpering, teething, and exhausted son. My eyes burning from fatigue, my muscles aching from holding him for hours on end (he's a wee bit bigger than the average one-year-old), I wiped a tear from David's face and reached for his blanket from the floor. He grabbed it and pulled it to his face and snuggled in closer against my chest.

I started knitting this blanket for David years earlier when he was merely a whisper in my consciousness. I stopped knitting when I first discovered I'm infertile and started again toward the end of my treatment. Someone told me then that I was knitting again because I was ready to become a mother (who knew it would still be years before motherhood would happen for me?).

I would knit the blanket for a few weeks when I felt strong and optimistic and put it away when it became a painful reminder of what I couldn't have. I lovingly fingered the lavender yarn and looked at the stitches, measuring (and then measuring again) to see how much more was required before I finished. Every stitch and click of my knitting needles articulated the inevitability of this moment, late at night, with my child in my arms. But I didn't anticipate how the stitches of this blanket would intertwine us.

The lavender blanket that soothed my fears and reassured me during my quest to become a mother has become David's lovey, his security against the challenges of babyhood. As he reached for it and wrapped himself in it last night, I realized I've never been happier or more fulfilled in my life.

This little boy was meant to be our son. I have no doubt about this. David couldn't come to us through my body, so he found a remarkable woman to give him life, love, and cherish him. When he came home, everything I've ever believed about faith and destiny—about my infertility—was reaffirmed a thousand times over. Without my infertility and everything it taught me, I would not have been mature or spiritually centered enough to be a part of the life of this remarkable soul who I now have the privilege of parenting. What sweet joy this is!

Our infertility takes us to a strange, dark place full of fear and failure and longing. But it offers us our greatest potential for growth. Sure, I feel angry and hurt and confused sometimes. I'd be dishonest if I didn't acknowledge how hard this all is, even now that I'm a mom. But I've grown in profound ways because of the anger, the hurt, the confusion, and the struggles I've endured to have my son.

One day Charlie and I were driving home from the clinic. I don't remember why we had been there that day (which is weird because I remember almost every moment of my infertility treatment as if I had a DVD player in my head with scene selection) but I distinctly remember being overwhelmed by a sense of peace and rightness. And then I looked at Charlie and said, "I'm infertile!" Charlie smiled. "No, really? You're infertile?" I smiled and laughed, "Hell yeah, I'm infertile!" I put my arms over my head in victory and screamed at the top of my lungs, *"I'm infertile!"* This is who I am. This is my blessing.

This experience has changed my life, and changed it for the better. It brought me this beautiful little boy wrapped in a lavender blanket and (now finally) sleeping in my arms.

# Appendix

## Menstrual/Ovulation Cycle and the Feedback Loop

Ovulation is a pretty cool thing. Your body has a continuous positive-negative feedback loop between and among your hypothalamus, pituitary, and ovaries. This feedback loop is extremely delicate (hence the coolness of it), and if even one part of it is even a little bit quirky (due to stress, exercise, or illness) your entire cycle can get screwed up and you might not achieve a pregnancy. While we commonly think of the menstrual cycle as beginning on the first day of our periods (and it does start then), for purposes of this discussion, I am going to start describing the cycle to you from right after ovulation.

As you go through the second half of your menstrual cycle, estrogen in your body causes the lining in your uterus to develop and progesterone tells the lining to become receptive to a fertilized egg. If fertilization doesn't occur or you fail to implant a fertilized embryo, your levels of estrogen and progesterone start to fall fairly quickly. When your estrogen and progesterone levels fall below a certain point, it causes the lining to break down and be shed in what we all know (and love so much) as our period. On the first day of your period—while you are mourning the loss of another chance to become pregnant—your body is already gearing up to ovulate again.

Once your period starts, your hypothalamus kicks into gear producing a hormone known as GnRH (gonadotropin releasing hormone). The release of GnRH by the hypothalamus tells your pituitary to start producing two more hormones, FSH (follicle stimulating hormone) and LH (luteinizing hormone). Your pituitary then releases the FSH, and to a lesser extent the LH, into your bloodstream. Your pituitary will store some of the LH for later use.

The release of FSH into the bloodstream triggers a bunch of follicles in your ovary (or even both ovaries) to start developing. As the follicles begin to grow, they start to produce estrogen (specifically, estradiol or E2). The E2 released by the follicles enters your bloodstream and travels back to your pituitary. This production of E2 initially triggers the pituitary to make even more FSH, which signals the follicles to keep growing (the positive-feedback portion of the loop). However, as the follicles continue to grow, one of them will start to produce more E2 than the others and become the dominant follicle (sometimes two or more follicles will become dominant). The increased level of E2 produced by the dominant follicle travels back to the pituitary, telling it to shut down the production of FSH (this is the negative-feedback portion of the loop).

As the FSH level in the blood lowers, the dominant follicle enters its final maturation stage. The follicle begins to enlarge as the egg contained within it matures. As the dominant follicle reaches maximum growth, the E2 level in your blood will peak. This high E2 level causes the pituitary to become very sensitive to the GnRH being produced by your hypothalamus. This sudden sensitivity to GnRH triggers your pituitary to release all its stored LH. The surge of LH into your bloodstream (what is detected by ovulation predictor kits) signals the dominant follicle to begin the process of releasing your egg. In a natural cycle, some women will ovulate the day of the LH surge, while others may take up to thirty-six hours or longer to release the egg from the follicle.

In contrast to the natural cycle described above, in an ovulation induction cycle (which occurs during both IUI and IVF cycles), your doctor gives you drugs that tell your hypothalamus and pituitary what to do and when to do it. In an IUI cycle, the drugs will work with your body to achieve a good, healthy ovulation of a few to perhaps as many as several eggs. In an IVF cycle, your body's own feedback loop will be suppressed, and the doctors will use drugs to control every aspect of the stimulation of the follicles. In both IUI and IVF cycles your doctor is seeking to achieve a form of superovulation or, as it is also known, controlled ovarian hyperstimulation. In an IVF cycle, however, a greater degree of stimulation is sought to produce a greater number of eggs. The same follicle-stimulating drugs may be used in both an IUI and an IVF cycle, but the dosages of the drugs will differ, as the response sought from your ovary in IUI cycles is different (less) than in an IVF cycle.

## Finding the Right RE and/or Laboratory

Questions about the lab:

- Is the clinic affiliated with or part of a research- or academic-based medical center like a hospital?

- Is the embryology lab located at the hospital?

- Is the embryologist an M.D. or a board-certified Ph.D., known in the industry as a high-complexity clinical laboratory director?

- Has the embryologist or andrologist been responsible for discovering or improving any techniques or technologies?

- Does s/he publish articles on the clinic's research?

- How often is the embryology lab cleaned?

- Who is the andrologist?

- How many IVF egg retrievals and embryo transfers does the clinic perform per week?

- How many embryos does the clinic transfer to a patient in your age group and/or with your medical condition?

- What types of procedures are available to your patients?

- How many frozen embryo transfers do they perform per year?

- What are the criteria for freezing eggs?

- What is the protocol for frozen embryo transfers (FETs)?

- Does the clinic do blastocyst transfers?

- What are the clinic's criteria for performing blastocyst transfers?

- How many blastocyst transfers do they perform per year?

Questions to ask your RE:

- Where did you go to medical school?

- Where did you do your residency; where did you train?

- Are you board certified?

- How long have you been practicing reproductive medicine?

- Have you published any articles?

- Do you give lectures? Do you travel frequently to give lectures?

- Do you have any specific expertise, for example treating endometriosis or polycystic ovarian syndrome?

- How many eggs do you seek to recruit for IVF patients?

- What percentage of your patients experience OHSS (ovarian hyperstimulation syndrome, discussed in greater detail in chapter 7)?

- What are your criteria for canceling a patient's cycle?

- How would you recommend I start treatment?

- What types of protocols do you use?

- What type of protocol would you recommend for me?

- What do you think my prognosis is?

- How much time on average do you allocate to your appointments with patients? How strictly do you follow this schedule?

- Do you prefer patients who ask detailed questions about treatment, diagnosis, or symptoms?

- Are you available by phone, fax, or E-mail?

- Do your nurses return emergency calls, or do you?

- What time of day do you usually return phone calls?

## Understanding Success Rates

Let's take a look at a sample chart on page 260, which I've adapted from the CDC's 1999 statistics (you can find the link to the specific stats from which I based this chart in the Resources section). Please note that 1999 is the most recent year (as of the time I'm writing this) with available statistics. When reading this chart, the far left column identifies the parameters for the statistic, and the top row identifies the age group of the women to whom the statistics apply. I've italicized the important terms in the description of the statistic (in the far left column) that you need to watch out for. This chart breaks down statistics for nondonor IVF cycles, frozen embryo cycles using nondonor frozen embryos, and donor IVF cycles using fresh and frozen embryos.

As you can see from reading down the first column of statistics in this chart, this clinic reported the cumulative success rate for 535 nondonor IVF cycles among women less than thirty-five years of age. It reported success both in terms of cumulative pregnancy (49 percent) and live birth (44.3 percent) rates. The live birth rate is roughly 5 percent lower than the overall pregnancy rate (you do your own math in this table to find out the miscarriage rate). It also reported the percentage of retrievals (50.7 percent) and transfers (53.7 percent) resulting in live births

| Type of Cycle | Age of Woman | Age of Woman | Age of Woman | Age of Woman |
|---|---|---|---|---|
| **Fresh Embryos from Nondonor Eggs** | <35 | 35–37 | 38–40 | 41–42 |
| Total Number of Cycles Performed | 535 | 352 | 342 | 209 |
| Percentage of *cycles* resulting in *pregnancies* | 49 | 38.9 | 36.8 | 25.4 |
| Percentage of *cycles* resulting in *live births* | 44.3 | 32.4 | 25.4 | 15.8 |
| Percentage of *retrievals* resulting in *live births* | 50.7 | 39.2 | 33 | 20.2 |
| Percentage of *transfers* resulting in *live births* | 53.7 | 41.3 | 34 | 20.8 |
| Percentage of cancellations | 12.7 | 17.3 | 22.8 | 22 |
| Average number of embryos transferred | 2.9 | 3.5 | 3.7 | 4 |
| Percentage of *pregnancies* with *twins* | 35.9 | 32.1 | 23.8 | 11.3 |
| Percentage of *pregnancies* with *triplets* | 12.6 | 13.9 | 7.1 | 5.7 |
| Percentage of *live births* having *multiple infants* | 45.6 | 42.1 | 31 | 15.2 |
| **Frozen Embryos from Nondonor Eggs** | | | | |
| Number of transfers | 92 | 36 | 32 | 21 |
| Percentage of transfers resulting in live births | 34.8 | 30.6 | 9.4 | 9.5 |
| Average number of embryos transferred | 3.2 | 3.3 | 3.6 | 3.6 |
| **Donor Eggs (all ages combined)** | **Fresh Embryos** | **Frozen Embryos** | | |
| Number of transfers | 92 | 26 | | |
| Percentage of transfers resulting in live births | 47.8 | 15.4 | | |
| Average number of embryos transferred | 2.8 | 3 | | |

and gave you the overall cancellation rate (12.7 percent). Forty-five percent of the pregnancies in this age group resulted in a live birth of multiple infants. This clinic also reported that it performed ninety-two frozen transfers using nondonor frozen embryos with a resulting live birth rate of 34.8 percent. Similarly it reported ninety-two transfers for all age groups using fresh (not frozen, that's the next column to the right) donor eggs with a live birth rate of 47.8 percent.

Once you've oriented yourself in a table like this, you can read the results for the next column for the next oldest age group, women between the ages of thirty-five and thirty-seven. In the second column of statistics in this chart, this clinic reported the cumulative success rate for 352 non-donor IVF cycles. It reported success both in terms of cumulative pregnancy (38.9 percent) and live birth (32.4 percent) rates. Doing relatively simple math, you can see the miscarriage rate was roughly 7 percent, 2 percent higher than in the younger age group. Forty-two percent of the live births in this age group had multiple infants, 3 percent lower than in the younger age group.

## Preparing the Syringe

So you're going to give yourself a shot. Oh, what fun! Don't worry, I promise it's easier than it seems right now, and soon you'll be a pro at it! Let's go step by step through the process of preparing your syringe and finding a spot for your injection.

### PREPARING AN INJECTION USING AMPULES (GLASS VIALS) OF MEDICATION
Step 1: Find a spot in your house where you'll have room to work. I always used the kitchen counter. I kept all my supplies in a large plastic container in a corner on my kitchen counter, and I designated that entire area as my shot zone.

Step 2: Clean the area you will be using with alcohol. I used to pour a little alcohol on the counter and wipe it up with paper towels.

Step 3: Wash your hands with antibacterial cleaner.

Step 4: *For sub-Q injections,* remove the small needle from the syringe using a twisting (not pulling) motion to release the needle. Set this needle aside as you will need it again later (Step 17). *For IM injections,* you may ignore Steps 4 and 5.

Step 5: Attach a long (usually 22-gauge) needle to your syringe. You will use this big needle to mix your meds. You will use the same twisting motion to attach the needle as you used to remove it.

Step 6: Hold the ampule containing the dilutent (liquid) in one hand between your thumb and index finger.

Step 7: Gently tap the top of the ampule to remove the liquid (if any) from the tip of the ampule.

Step 8: Fold a paper towel into quarters or take a large gauze pad folded in half (I found that the little gauze pads tend to be too small to really protect you as you break the top off the ampule). Find the dot at the top of the ampule and face it *away from you.*

Step 9: Firmly snap the top/tip of the ampule away from you. It should break off in one neat piece (it's okay if the edge is a little jagged, and don't worry about getting glass shards in the syringe; the hole in your needle is much too small for glass ever to get sucked up inside the syringe). Throw away the paper towel and the top of the ampule.

Step 10: Place the long needle inside the ampule with the dilutent and pull the plunger of the syringe back until you have filled the syringe with 1 cc (or 1 ml) of dilutent from the ampule.

Step 11: Invert the syringe and needle so the needle points up to the ceiling. Gently tap the side of the syringe to get any air bubbles to float up to the top (near the needle).

Step 12: *Gently and slowly* depress the plunger (with the needle pointing up toward the ceiling) to push the air bubbles out of the needle. When you see a tiny drop of liquid at the top of the needle you know you have removed the air bubbles.

Step 13: Check the measurement in the syringe to make sure you still have 1 cc of dilutent in the syringe. The top ridge of the plunger should be at the 1 cc (1 ml) mark. If you don't, you may need to open another ampule of dilutent to add some more liquid until you've got 1 cc in your syringe. If you've got 1 cc of dilutent in your syringe, carefully place the cap on the needle and lay the syringe down on the sterile countertop or work space while you open the ampules of medication. I don't recommend opening all the ampules at the beginning, as it is too easy to knock one of them over and spill the precious powdered medication.

Step 14: Take out the number of ampules containing powdered medication that you'll need to mix in your dilutent. For example, if you're on 3FSH you're going to need three ampules of medication. (Ask your nurse if you have any questions about how many ampules to use, especially if they are changing your dosage instructions!) Repeat the same procedure (Steps 8 and 9) for breaking the ampules that are filled with your (powdered) medication.

Step 15: Remove the cap from the syringe and slowly inject the dilutent into the first ampule of medicine. Remove the syringe when you're finished, place the cap on, and place the capped syringe on your countertop.

Step 16: Gently rotate the ampule between your thumb and forefinger (or the palms of your hand) to mix the medication and dilutent. *Do not shake* the ampule. When the liquid is clear (it may take a few seconds) you've correctly mixed the medication.

Step 17: Following Step 10, withdraw the medication from the ampule and inject the liquid into the next ampule of medication (you will use the same liquid each time you mix your medication for this injection). Repeat Step 16 to mix the medication. Repeat Steps 16 and 17 until all your ampules of medication have been mixed with the dilutent.

Step 18: Carefully draw back the plunger on the syringe to draw the liquid medication down out of the needle and away from the top of the syringe (you need a buffer of air when you change the needles so as not to lose medication). Carefully replace the cap on the needle and twist the needle to remove it from the syringe. *For sub-Q injections,* replace the small needle you removed in the beginning (Step 4) onto the syringe using a twisting motion. *For IM injections,* you can use the same 22-gauge needle that you used to mix your medications (or you may place a new

22-gauge needle on the syringe if you want to be sure to have the sharpest needle going into your tush).

Step 19: *For sub-Q injections,* locate a spot on your body to do your injection and wipe it down with some alcohol. Allow the alcohol to dry.

Step 20: Follow the instructions in Step 12 to remove any air and/or air bubbles from the syringe.

Step 21: Hold the syringe in your dominant hand (if you're a righty, this would be your right hand) and use the other hand to pinch a fold of skin at the site you've selected to do your shot.

Step 22: Carefully but quickly insert the needle into the middle of the pinched fold of skin. No dartlike motion here, just be definitive and swift! It won't hurt too much, I promise!

Step 23: Slowly depress the plunger at a steady rate until all the medication has been injected.

Step 24: Remove the needle by pulling it out of the pinched fold using a straight motion (don't pull it out at an angle, it will hurt if you do!).

Step 25: Place the syringe on the counter and place a clean gauze pad over the injection site; rub or massage gently to help the medication absorb into your tissue. If need be, place a bandage over the injection site.

Step 26: Recap your syringe and place it in a Sharps container (this is a sterile safe needle disposal container, usually provided by your pharmacy. If not, use a wide-topped plastic container and dispose of your needles at your clinic).

Step 27: *For IM injections,* locate a spot on your tush to do your injection. Wipe it down with an alcohol-soaked pad and allow the alcohol to dry. I recommend lying down for this injection, but you may also sit (if you're doing it yourself) or stand (relaxing into the hip on the opposite side where you will be doing the injection and allowing your knee to bend slightly on the side where the needle will go in).

Step 28: Hold the syringe in your dominant hand like a pencil (if you're a righty, this is your right hand). Using your other hand, gently stretch the skin at the injection site to help the needle go in without tension.

Step 29: Insert the needle at a ninety-degree angle; using a straight motion, quickly insert the needle.

Step 30: Use one hand to stabilize the syringe and use your other hand to slowly draw back slightly on the plunger and watch for blood (this is pretty rare). It is normal to feel resistance or see an air bubble. You do not want to pull back so much that you withdraw fluid from your muscle. If you don't see any blood, the needle is correctly inserted into the muscle. If you do see blood, withdraw the needle and cover the injection site with a gauze pad and apply light pressure to stop the bleeding. Discard the syringe and medication and start all over again with a fresh syringe and new medication.

Step 31: Depress the plunger slowly and steadily.

Step 32: When all the medication has been injected, carefully remove the needle using a straight motion (you don't want to remove the needle at an angle; this hurts).

Step 33: Place the syringe on the counter (or bedside table), place a clean gauze pad over the injection site, and rub or massage gently to help the medication absorb into your tissue. If need be, place a bandage over the injection site.

Step 34: Recap your syringe and place it in a Sharps container (this is a sterile safe needle disposal container, usually provided by your pharmacy. If not, use a wide-topped plastic container and dispose of your needles at your clinic).

Congratulations! Go do something good to reward yourself (chick flick, good dinner, back rub from your hubby).

### PREPARING AN INJECTION USING VIALS (GLASS BOTTLES WITH CAPS) OF MEDICATION

Step 1: Open each vial by removing the plastic top. Wipe the rubber top of each vial with an alcohol-soaked pad to remove germs.

Step 2: Clean the area you will be using with alcohol. I used to pour a little alcohol on the counter and wipe it up with paper towels.

Step 3: Wash your hands with antibacterial cleaner.

Step 4: *For sub-Q injections,* remove the small needle from the syringe using a twisting (not pulling) motion to release the needle. Set this needle aside as you will need it again later (Step 13). *For IM injections,* you will use the long (22-gauge) needle on your syringe for mixing your medication and later (Step 13) replace it with a new fresh, sharp, 22-gauge needle. *For IM Injections,* you may skip Step 5.

Step 5: Attach a long (usually 22-gauge) needle to your syringe. You will use this big needle to mix your meds. You will use the same twisting motion to attach the needle as you used to remove it.

Step 6: Draw 1 cc (1 ml) of air into the syringe by pulling back on the plunger to the 1 cc (1 ml) mark. Inject this air into the vial containing liquid (hold the vial on your countertop) by sticking the needle into the center of the rubber stopper at the top of the vial and depressing the plunger. This will give you additional suction when removing the liquid from the vial.

Step 7: Invert the vial and syringe (the needle is still attached to the vial), holding the vial in your left or nondominant hand and the syringe in your right or dominant hand. Carefully bring the needle down so it is below the liquid level and is completely surrounded by fluid.

Step 8: Carefully pull the plunger down to withdraw slightly more than 1 cc (1 ml) of liquid from the vial and remove the needle from the vial.

Step 9: *Gently and slowly* depress the plunger (with the needle pointing up toward the ceiling) to push the air bubbles out of the needle. When you see a tiny drop of liquid at the top of the needle, you know you have removed the air bubbles. Check to make sure you've got 1 cc (1 ml) of fluid in the syringe (the top ridge of the plunger should be at the 1 cc (1 ml) mark.

Step 10: Inject the 1 cc (1 ml) of dilutent into the vial of powdered medication. You may remove the needle for the next step or leave it in, depending on which is easier for you.

Step 11: Gently rotate the vial between your thumb and forefinger (or the palms of your hand) to mix the medication and dilutent. *Do not shake* the vial. When the liquid is clear (it may take a few seconds), you've correctly mixed the medication. Repeat Steps 10 and 11 to mix each vial of medication you need (you use the same dilutent every time you mix a new vial of medication).

Step 12: With the needle in the vial, invert the vial and syringe so that your needle is pointing up toward the ceiling and your vial is upside down. Pull the needle down below the liquid level and make sure it's surrounded completely by fluid. Carefully pull down on the plunger until you've removed all the liquid from the vial and remove the needle from the vial.

Step 13: Carefully draw back the plunger on the syringe to draw the liquid medication down out of the needle and away from the top of the syringe (you need a buffer of air when you change the needles so as not to lose medication). Carefully replace the cap on the needle and twist the needle to remove it from the syringe. *For sub-Q injections,* replace the small needle you removed in the beginning (Step 4) onto the syringe using a twisting motion. *For IM injections,* take a fresh long needle (22-gauge) and place the needle on the syringe using a twisting motion (you will need a fresh, sharp needle to do the injection; the needle you were using is now very dull from being injected into the rubber cap at the top of the vial).

Step 14: *For sub-Q injections,* locate a spot on your body to do your injection and wipe it down with some alcohol. Allow the alcohol to dry.

Step 15: Follow the instructions in Step 9 to remove any air and/or air bubbles from the syringe.

Step 16: Hold the syringe in your dominant hand (if you're a righty, this would be your right hand) and use the other hand to pinch a fold of skin at the site you've selected to do your shot.

Step 17: Carefully but quickly insert the needle into the middle of the pinched fold of skin. No dartlike motion here, just be definitive and swift! It won't hurt too much, I promise!

Step 18: Slowly depress the plunger at a steady rate until all the medication has been injected.

Step 19: Remove the needle by pulling it out of the pinched fold using a straight motion (don't pull it out at an angle, it will hurt if you do!).

Step 20: Place the syringe on the counter and place a clean gauze pad over the injection site, rubbing or massaging gently to help the medication absorb into your tissue. If need be, place a bandage over the injection site.

Step 21: Recap your syringe and place it in a Sharps container (this is a sterile safe needle disposal container, usually provided by your pharmacy. If not, use a wide-topped plastic container and dispose of your needles at your clinic).

Step 22: *For IM injections,* locate a spot on your tush to do your injection. Wipe it down with an alcohol-soaked pad and allow the alcohol to dry. I recommend lying down for this injection, but you may also sit (if you're doing it yourself) or stand (relaxing into the hip on the opposite side where you will be doing the injection and allowing your knee to bend slightly on the side where the needle will go in).

Step 23: Hold the syringe in your dominant hand like a pencil (if you're a righty, this is your right hand). Using your other hand, gently stretch the skin at the injection site to help the needle go in without tension.

Step 24: Insert the needle at a ninety-degree angle; using a straight motion, quickly insert the needle.

Step 25: Use one hand to stabilize the syringe and use your other hand to slowly draw back slightly on the plunger and watch for blood (this is pretty rare). It is normal to feel resistance or see an air bubble. You do not want to pull back so much that you withdraw fluid from your muscle. If you don't see any blood, the needle is correctly inserted into the muscle. If you do see blood, withdraw the needle and cover the injection site with a gauze pad and apply light pressure to stop the bleeding. Discard the syringe and medication and start all over again with a fresh syringe and new medication.

Step 26: Depress the plunger slowly and steadily.

Step 27: When all the medication has been injected, carefully remove the needle using a straight motion (you don't want to remove the needle at an angle; this hurts).

Step 28: Place the syringe on the counter (or bedside table), place a clean gauze pad over the injection site, and rub or massage gently to help the medication absorb into your tissue. If need be, place a bandage over the injection site.

Step 29: Recap your syringe and place it in a Sharps container (this is a sterile safe needle disposal container, usually provided by your pharmacy. If not, use a wide-topped plastic container and dispose of your needles at your clinic).

Congratulations! Go do something good to reward yourself (chick flick, good dinner, back rub from your hubby).

### SOME TIPS ON INJECTING PROGESTERONE IN OIL

Before preparing your syringe you will want to warm the vial of oil slightly to help the medication be injected. You can warm the vial by placing it in your bra or under your arm for ten to fifteen minutes. Follow the steps above for preparing your syringe for an IM injection (note that you don't have to mix the medication or introduce air into the vial for more suction). Make sure to wipe the top of the rubber stopper down with alcohol as it has been under your arm or in your bra and exposed to germs! Before doing this injection, I recommend lying on a reusable ice pack to chill and slightly numb the area where you will do the injection. After performing the injection, place a bandage over the injection site and then lie on a heating pad for ten to fifteen minutes to help warm your muscle and facilitate the absorption of the progesterone (I use the Band-Aid to help mark the spot to warm with the heating pad).

### SOME TIPS ON INJECTING HEPARIN OR LOVENOX

Ice the injection spot thoroughly before and after performing the injection. This will reduce discomfort, stinging, and bruising from the injection. Apply steady pressure to the injection site after performing the shot, but *do not* massage the area (this will increase your bruising).

These injections can be quite painful and can cause a lot of bruising. If need be, talk to your doctor about using a super small-gauge needle (insulin needles or even smaller, 30-gauge needles). The Lovenox comes preloaded in glass syringes. If you want to use a smaller needle than what comes with the preloaded syringe (I found this helped to reduce pain from the injection), you can remove the needle from a standard 3 cc (3 ml) syringe, draw back on the plunger to the 1 cc mark, inject the Lovenox into the 3 cc (3 ml) syringe, and then place your smaller-gauge needle on this syringe. Don't forget to follow the steps to remove air and air bubbles from the syringe before performing the injection!

## ICSI, Embryos, and Blastocysts

I found it really useful when I was going through a cycle to be able to look at pictures to help me understand what doctors were describing. On the following pages I'm giving you pictures of what ICSI (intracytoplasmic sperm injection) looks like as it is being performed, what cleaving (dividing and growing) embryos look like between fertilization and day 3 after fertilization, and what blastocysts look like.

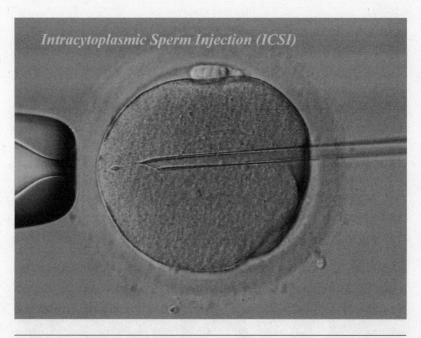

*Intracytoplasmic Sperm Injection (ICSI)*

The funny-looking thing on the left of the image is the pipette that is holding the egg in place. The long skinny thing that extends from the right side of the image into the egg is the needle that is injecting the sperm. To the far left of the egg you can see the tiny sperm that was injected.

## Cleaving Embryos

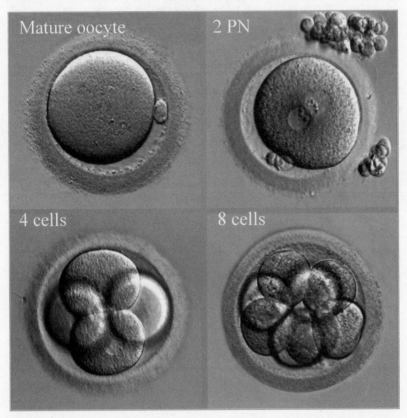

Mature oocyte

2 PN

4 cells

8 cells

These pictures show the process of an egg going from a single cell to a day-3 embryo. The first image is a mature egg, the second image on the top right is a fertilized egg that has two pronuclei (2PN) and is cleaving (dividing), the third image on the lower left is a day-2 four-celled embryo, and the last image on the bottom right is a day-3 eight-celled embryo.

## Blastocysts

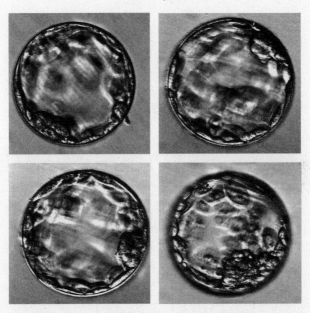

These images are of embryos that have reached the blastocyst stage of development, approximately five days after fertilization.

# Resources

## CHAPTER 3

**RESOLVE**
1310 Broadway
Somerville, MA 02144
(617) 623-0744
*www.Resolve.org*
*info@resolve.org*

RESOLVE has a national help line
(888) 623-0744
It's open Monday through Friday, 9
A.M. to noon and 1 P.M. to 4 P.M. eastern time and Monday evenings from 7
P.M. to 11 P.M.

RESOLVE has a national Medical
help line
(888) 623-0744
A registered nurse who can help you
understand your treatment plan and
formulate questions to ask your doctor
staffs the Medical help line. Medical
Call-In is available to members only, on
Wednesdays from 1 P.M. to 4 P.M. eastern time.

**American Infertility Association**
666 Fifth Avenue, Suite 278
New York, NY 10103
(718) 621-5083
*www.americaninfertility.org*
*info@americaninfertility.org*

Help line for referrals and support
(888) 917-3777
Mon–Fri. 10 A.M.–3 P.M. EST
Tues., 5 A.M.–10 P.M. EST

**American Society for Reproductive Medicine**
1209 Montgomery Highway
Birmingham, AL 35216-2809
(205) 978-5000
*www.asrm.org*

**The Society for Assisted Reproductive Technology**
Joyce Zeitz, Executive Administrator
1209 Montgomery Highway
Birmingham, AL 35216
(205) 978-5000 X109
*www.sart.org*
*jzeitz@asrm.org*

Centers for Disease Control—IVF
Statistics
CDC's Reproductive Health
Information Source
Assisted Reproductive Technology
Reports
*www.cdc.gov/nccdphp/drh/art.htm*

## CHAPTER 4

### Reproductive Immunologists

Carolyn B. Coulam, M.D.
Medical Director
Sher Institute for Reproductive
Medicine
233 E. Erie, Suite 500
Chicago, IL 60611
(312) 573-1900
*www.haveababy.com*
*chicago@haveababy.com*

Alan E. Beer, M.D.
Reproductive Medicine Program
Finch University of Health Science
Chicago Medical School
3333 Green Bay Road
North Chicago, IL 60064
(847) 578-3233
*www.repro-med.net*
*info@repro-med.net*

Reproductive Immunology Associates
6850 Sepulveda Blvd., Suite 210
Van Nuys, CA 91405
(818) 781-5195
*www.rialab.com*
*info@rialab.com*

The InterNational Council on
Infertility Information Dissemination,
Inc.
*www.inciid.org/interinfertility.html*
(Search under Immune Issues, Miscar-
riage, and Reproductive Failure.)

Early Path Medical Consultation
Services
(Pathology Services Working for Safer
Pregnancies)
Carolyn M. Salafia, M.D.
86 Edgewood Avenue
Larchmont, NY 10538
(914) 834-2598
*www.earlypath.com/earlypath/intro.html*

Recurrent pregnancy loss information
*www.fertilityplus.org/faq/miscarriage/*
*resources.html#web*

## CHAPTER 5

Oxford Endometriosis Gene Study
(OXEGENE)
The OXEGENE Study
Nuffield Department of Obstetrics &
Gynecology
University of Oxford
The Research Institute
Churchill Hospital
OXFORD OX3 7LJ
United Kingdom
Fax: +44 1865 769141
Tel: +44 1865 225856
(Leave a message on the answering
machine, and a member of the
research team will return your call.)

*http://www.medicine.ox.ac.uk/ndog/*
*oxegene/oxegene.htm*
*oxegene@obs-gyn.ox.ac.uk*

**The Center for Uterine Fibroids**
Brigham and Women's Hospital
Departments of Obstetrics/
Gynecology and Pathology
623 Thorn Building
20 Shattuck Street
Boston, MA 02115
(800) 722-5520 X80081
*http://www.fibroids.net*

**Books on Endometriosis:**

*Endometriosis: A Practical Guide to*
*Healing Through Nutrition*
Dian Mills, M.A. and Michael
Vernon, Ph.D., HCLD
Element ©2001

*Endometriosis, Infertility & Traditional*
*Chinese Medicine: A Laywoman's Guide*
Bob Flaws
Blue Poppy Press ©1989

**CHAPTER 6**

**Center for Male Reproductive**
**Medicine and Microsurgery**
The New York Hospital–Cornell
Medical Center
525 E. 68th Street
New York, NY 10021
*www.maleinfertility.com*

**Marc Goldstein, M.D.**
(212) 746-5470
*http://www.inciid.org/advisory/*
*mgoldstein.html*

**Peter N. Schlegel, M.D.**
(212) 746-5491
*http://www.inciid.org/members/*
*schlegel.html*

**See also:**
*www.inciid.org/directory-urology.html*

**CHAPTER 7**

**Adoption Books**

*Adopting After Infertility*
Patricia Irwin Johnston
Perspectives Press ©1992
(Expect to cry when you read this
book!)

*The Long Awaited Stork: A Guide to*
*Parenting After Infertility*
Ellen Sarasohn Glazer
Jossey-Bass ©1998
(Discusses third-party parenting
arrangements in addition to adoption.)

*Launching a Baby's Adoption: Practical*
*Strategies for Parents and Professionals*
Patricia Irwin Johnston
Perspectives Press ©1997

*Adoption Without Fear*
James L. Gritter, MSW, Ed.
Corona ©1989
(Somewhat outdated, but provides an
excellent look at open adoption.)

*Adoption Is a Family Affair: What
Relatives and Friends Must Know*
Patricia Irwin Johnston
Perspectives Press ©2001

*Adoption Journeys: Parents Tell Their
Stories*
Carole S. Turner, Ed.
McBooks Press ©1999
(Wonderful, heartwarming stories of
all types of adoption; international,
domestic, and single-parent.)

**Other Good Resources on Adoption**

*Adoptive Families Magazine*
*www.adoptivefamilies.com/index.php*

The Gladney Center for Adoption
*www.adoptionsbygladney.com*

A great adoption website for getting
familiar with adoption:
*www.adoption.com*

**Gestational Surrogacy**

*A Matter of Trust: The Guide to
Gestational Surrogacy*
Gail Dutton
Clouds Publishing ©1997

**Alternative Treatments**

*Inconceivable: Winning the Fertility Game*
Julia Indichova
Adell Press ©1997

*The Whole Person Fertility Program: A
Revolutionary Mind-Body Process to Help
You Conceive*
Nirvani B. Payne, M.S.
Three Rivers Press © 1997

*The Infertility Diet: Get Pregnant and
Prevent Miscarriage*
Fern Reiss
PBJ Press ©1999

*Getting Pregnant Naturally: Healthy
Choices to Boost Your Chances of
Conceiving Without Fertility Drugs*
Winifred Conkling
Avon ©1999

*Taking Charge of Your Fertility: The
Definitive Guide to Natural Birth Control
and Pregnancy Achievement*
Toni Weshcler, MPH
Harper Perennial ©1995

*Endometriosis: A Practical Guide to Healing
Through Nutrition*
Dian Mills, M.A. and Michael
Vernon, Ph.D., HCLD
Element ©2001

*Endometriosis, Infertility & Traditional
Chinese Medicine: A Laywoman's Guide*
Bob Flaws
Blue Poppy Press ©1989

**Mind/Body Work**

Alice D. Domar, Ph.D., Director
Mind/Body Center for Women's
Health
Boston IVF

Waltham, MA
(781) 434–6500
*www.bostonivf.com*

**Mind/Body Medical Institute**
Chestnut Hill, MA
(866) 509–0732
(617) 991–0102
*www.mbmi.org*

**The Center for Reproductive Medicine and Infertility**
Cornell University
Weill Medical College
505 East 70th Street
New York, NY 10021
(212) 746–1745
*www.ivf.org*

**Mind/Body Institute**
Los Angeles, CA
(213) 688–6119
*www.mindbodyinfertility.com*

**Living Child-Free**

*Reconceiving Women: Separating Motherhood From Female Identity*
Mardy Ireland, Ph.D.
Guilford Press ©1993

*Without Child: Challenging the Stigma of Childlessness*
Laurie Lisle
Routledge ©1999

*The Childless Revolution*
Madelyn Cain
Perseus © 2002

**Embryo Donation**

*The Long Awaited Stork: A Guide to Parenting After Infertility*
Ellen Sarasohn Glazer
Jossey-Bass ©1998

**RESOLVE**
Free fact sheet on Embyro Donation and directory of clinics offering embryo donation services by state.
(617) 623–6222 or
*www.resolve.org*

**Society for Assisted Reproductive Technology**
(205) 978–5000 x109
*www.sart.org*
*jzeitz@asrm.org*

See also:
*www.perspectivespress.com/carembryo.html*
*www.fertilityplus.org/faq/donor.html#embryo*

**CHAPTER 9**

**ARC**
Advanced Reproductive Care, Inc.
540 University Avenue, Suite 250
Palo Alto, CA 94301
*www.arcfertility.com*
*info@arcfertility.com*

**IntegraMed America Inc.**
1 Manhattanville Rd.
Purchase, NY 10577
(914) 253–8000
(800) 458–0044
*www.integramed.com/*
*info@integramed.com*

**Family Fee Plan**
225 Turnpike Road
Southborough, MA 01772
(866) 733-3373
*www.amerifee.com/fertility-financing/*
*index.asp*
*ffp@feeplan.com*

**IVF Meds—On-line Pharmacies**

**Apthorp Pharmacy**
(800) 775-3582
Fax prescriptions toll free to (877)
846-6031 with name, telephone
number, and prescription info. Ship
by FedEx overnight or same-day
messenger.
2201 Broadway (78th Street)
New York, NY 10024
*www.apthorp.com*
*info@apthorp.com*

See also:
*www.fertilitymeds.com*
*www.ivpcare.com/Infertility/infertility.asp*
*www.freedomdrug.com*
*www.fertilityneighbor.com*

**Infertility as a Disability**
(An analysis of disability law as it may
apply to infertility.)
*www.inciid.org/bragdon-abbott.html*

## CHAPTER 13

HCG levels broken down by singleton
and multiple pregnancies
*www.advancedfertility.com/earlypre.htm*

## CHAPTER 14
### Adoptive Breastfeeding

The Adoptive Breastfeeding Resource
Web site (for adoptive moms and those
using gestational surrogates)

*www.fourfriends.com/ubbthreads/*
*categories.php?Cat=*

The Newman-Goldfarb Induced
Lactation Protocol and general
information
*www.asklenore.com/*

*Breastfeeding the Adopted Baby, rev. ed.*
Debra Stewart Peterson
Corona © 1994

# Index

Page numbers in *italic* indicate illustrations; those in **bold** indicate tables.

Academic-based medical center, 42

Acquired blood-clotting disorder, 93

Acquired thrombophilias, 60, 61

Activated partial thromboplastin time (APTT), 62

Acupuncture, 11, 92, 126, 127, 217–218

Addictiveness of treatment, 247–248

Adhesions, 71–72

Admission policies and success, 51–52

Adoption, 119–125. *See also* Decisions about options

agency adoption, 119, 121, 122–124

authenticity issues, 122

background of mother and, 121

birth parent issues, 121, 123

closed adoption, 121, 122, 131

costs for, 120, 123–124

domestic adoption, 119, 121

Elizabeth Swire Falker's story, xix, xviii, xxi, 1, 19, 20–21

embryo donation, 131–132, 146, 279

facilitator adoption, 119, 125

flexibility for, 121

foster care adoption, 125

gender of baby and, 121

international adoption, 119, 121, 124

misconceptions about, 117

mother's background and, 121

older couples and, 124

open adoption, 121–122, 129

parenting right of birth mother, 123

private attorney adoption, 119, 121, 122–124

referrals for, 125

relinquishment laws, 123

reputation of agencies, 125

resources for, 277–278, 279, 280

risk level, 123, 125, 132

same-sex couples and, 124

semiopen adoption, 121, 122

wait time, 121

"Advanced maternal age," 4, 91, 97, 140

Advanced Reproductive Care (ARC), 169, 173

Advocacy, 180–184

clinic, working with, 182

consumer business of reproductive medicine, 31, 34, 47, 182

cycle paperwork, having, 181

education about diagnosis, 182

enemies at clinic, avoiding, 183

medical records, knowledge of, 181

mistakes, avoiding, 118, 147, 180–181

standing up for yourself, 183–184

steps of treatment, knowing, 181–182

venting, avoiding, 183

Affording infertility. *See* Financial aspects of infertility

African American women and fibroids, 80

"Age, advanced maternal," 4, 91, 97, 140

Age and shared-risk programs, 169, 170

Agency adoption, 119, 121, 122–124

Aggressiveness

of reproductive endocrinologists (REs), 46–47

of shared-risk programs, 173

Agreeing with comment-maker, 154–155

Alternative (holistic) therapies, 98, 125–127, 278–279

American Infertility Association (AIA), 32, 33, 100, 141, 219
American Society for Reproductive Medicine (ASRM), 32, 33, 48, 50, 100, 132, 141
Ampules, preparing injection using, 261–265
ANA (antinuclear antibodies), 61, 62
Anatomical issues, male, 107–109
Androgen blood test, 57
Andrologists, 41, 42, 43
Antagon, **188,** 190, 192
Antibody problems, 60, 61–63
Antinuclear antibodies (ANA), 61, 62
Antiphospholipid antibodies (APA), 61–62, 93
Antithyroid antibodies, 61, 62
Apthorp Pharmacy, 178, 280
APTT (activated partial thromboplastin time), 62
ARC (Advanced Reproductive Care), 169, 173
ASRM (American Society for Reproductive Medicine), 32, 33, 48, 50, 100, 132, 141
Assisted hatching, 44, 47, 227
Assisted reproductive technologies (ART), xxi, 7. *See also* Intrauterine insemination (IUI); In vitro fertilization (IVF); Surviving infertility roller coaster
Audited statistics of clinics, 48
Authenticity issues, adoption, 122
Azoospermia, 102, 111–113

Baby-killing cells, 60, 63–64, 95–97
Baby showers, 156–157
Background of mother and adoption, 121
Basal body temperature (BBT), 1–2
BCPs (birth control pills), 76, 192–193
Beginning treatment, 200–235. *See also* Cycle, understanding your; Monitoring treatment
assisted hatching, 44, 47, 227
blastocyst stage of embryo, 223, 224, 225, 226, *273*
blastocyst transfer, 224–227
blastomeres, 223
care package, creating, 204–205
cleaving (dividing) of embryos, 223, *272*
culture mediums with in vitro fertilization (IVF), 225
cycle day 3 (CD3), 200–201, 207–208
cycle day 7/9 (CD7/9), 208
day-3 transfer, 224, 226
day-5 transfer, 224, 225, 226, 227
embryo and in vitro fertilization (IVF), 228–230
embryo quality, 223–227

embryo transfer, 203, 222–223, 228–230
failed cycles, 222, 242
financial planning, 201
fragmentation, 223–224
frozen embryo transfers (FET), 15–16, 17, 44, 230–233
human chorionic gonadotropin (HCG), **188,** 190, 195, 207, 208, 212, 214–215
implantation, 11–12, 234
implantation spotting, 233–234
intrauterine insemination (IUI), 201–202, 206, 219–220
in vitro fertilization (IVF), 201, 202–203, 206, 220–223, 228–230
monitoring, 207–208, 208–209
patient coordinators, 202
pregnancy signs, 233–234
pregnancy test, 235
"pregnancy worthy" embryos, 231
program FET, 231–232
resting during in vitro fertilization (IVF), 203
retrieval (oocyte retrieval), 203, 220–222
scheduling cycle, 200–204
sensitivity of body and, 206–207
stress and, 202, 203–204, 207
two-week wait, 229, 233–235
wait list for cycle, 202
zona pellucida (shell) of embryo, 223, 227
Benefits of infertility, xviii–xix, 253–254
Beta HCG test, 12, 14, 15, 236, 237–240, **240**
Big vs. small clinics, 40–41
Biofeedback techniques, 126
Birth control pills (BCPs), 76, 192–193
Birth defects and ICSI, 106–107
Birth parent issues, adoption, 121, 123
Blastocyst stage of embryo, 223, 224, 225, 226, *273*
Blastocyst transfer
clinic rates, 51
day-6 transfer, 224–227
multiple births and, 146
reproductive endocrinologists (REs) and, 44–45
Blastomeres, 223
Blood-clotting disorders (thrombophilias), 12, 60–61, 93–94
Blood tests, 55–64, 56–64. *See also* Invasive tests
acquired thrombophilias, 60, 61
activated partial thromboplastin time (APTT), 62
androgen blood test, 57
antibody problems, 60, 61–63

antinuclear antibodies (ANA), 61, 62
antiphospholipid antibodies (APA), 61–62, 93
antithyroid antibodies, 61, 62
baby-killing cells, 60, 63–64, 95–97
blood-clotting disorders (thrombophilias), 12,
    60–61, 93–94
cytogenic analysis, 58
cytokines, 63–64, 95
dilation and curettage (D & C), 58, 59, 64
egg quality, 56–57, 87, 88–92, 212–213
embryo toxicity assay (ETA), 64
estradiol (E2), 56–57, 88, 89–91
follicle-stimulating hormone (FSH), 56–57,
    88–89, 90–91
genetic karyotyping, 58–59, 110
human leukocyte antigens (HLA), 63, 95–97
hyperhomocysteinemia, 12, 61
immune testing, 12, 59–64, 93–97
inherited thrombophilias, 60–61
in vitro fertilization (IVF) failure, 58–64
lab specific tests, 56–57
Leiden factor V mutation R560Q, 61
lupuslike anticoagulant antibodies, 61, 62
luteinizing hormone (LH), 56–57, 215
MTHFR gene, 12, 13, 16, 61, 93
natural killer (NK) cells, 63, 95
ovulation, 2–3, 4, 56, 57, 84–87
polycystic ovarian syndrome (PCOS), 57, 84–
    87
preimplantation genetic diagnosis (PGD), 58–
    59, 107, 140–141
prolactin blood test, 57
protein C or S abnormalities, 61
prothrombin gene mutation 20210 (GA), 61
recurrent pregnancy loss, 58–64, 93–97
reproductive immunophenotype test (RIP),
    63
resources for, 276
serum progesterone blood test, 56
sperm analysis, 102
tumor necrosis factor (TNF), 63
Board certification, 30, 42
Boost protocol, 191, 192
Bosses, telling about infertility, 153
Buddy for cycle, 198
Business of reproductive medicine, 31, 34, 47,
    182
"Buyer beware," 34

Canceling cycle, 211
Cancellation criteria for patient's cycle, 46
Career decisions, 6–7, 8

Care package, creating, 204–205
Categories of friends, 151–153
Caucasian women and fibroids, 80
CAV (vas deferens malformation), 102, 108–109
Celebrating pregnancy, 241–242
Center for Reproductive Medicine and
    Infertility (CRMI), 5, 7, 11, 17–18
Center for Uterine Fibroids (Brigham and
    Women's Hospital), 80
Centers for Disease Control (CDC), 48, 50
Checklist, insurance, 167–168
Chemical pregnancy rates, 49, 50
Child-free living, 127–128, 279
"Chocolate cyst" (endometrioma), 75
Chung, Pak H.
    beginning treatment, 207, 233
    Elizabeth Swire Falker's story, 7, 8, 9, 10, 11,
        12, 13, 14, 15, 16, 18, 19
    ovarian hyperstimulation syndrome (OHSS)
        risk, 147
    reproductive endocrinologist (RE), finding,
        35, 147, 207, 233, 242
    success of cycle, 242
Cleaning of embryology lab, 43
Clean slate, starting with (Rule #1), 23–25, 29
Cleaving (dividing) of embryos, 223, 272
Climara, **188**
Clinic, working with (advocacy), 182
Clinical pregnancy rates, 49, 50
Clinic evaluation, 40–45, 257–258. See also
    Reproductive endocrinologist (RE),
    finding
    academic-based medical center, 42
    andrologists, 41, 42, 43
    big vs. small clinics, 40–41
    blastocyst transfers, 44–45
    cleaning of embryology lab, 43
    coculture program, 44
    egg management importance, 41
    embryologists, 41, 42, 43
    embryology lab, 42, 43
    embryo transfer policies, 43
    freezing eggs criteria, 44
    frozen embryo transfers (FETs), 44
    number of procedures performed weekly/
        yearly, 43, 44, 45
    procedures available at clinic, 44
    research-based medical center, 42
    small vs. big clinics, 40–41
    sperm management importance, 41
    success rates, comparing, 51–52

Clomid, 26, 69, 83, 133, 187, **188,** 189, 190, 196
Clomid challenge test, 90, 91
Closed adoption, 121, 122, 131
"Coasting," 210
COBRA (Consolidated Omnibus Budget Reconciliation Act), 176
Coculture program, 44
Comparisons to others, avoiding, 209
Compassionate doctors, 32, 35
Condescending suggestions, 154
Confronting comment-maker, 155–156
Consolidated Omnibus Budget Reconciliation Act (COBRA), 176
Consumer business of reproductive medicine, 31, 34, 47, 182
Controlled ovarian hyperstimulation, 186
Costs. *See also* Financial aspects of infertility
 adoption, 120, 123–124
 decisions about options and, 118–119
 infertility workup, 160–161
Coulam, Carolyn, 19, 96
Credit cards for infertility payment, 175
Cryomyolysis, 82
Cryopreserving (freezing)
 of embryos, 146
 of sperm, 113
Culture mediums, IVF, 225
Cycle, understanding your, 185–199. *See also* Beginning treatment; Medications
 boost protocol, 191, 192
 buddy for, 198
 cycle day 2 (CD2), 192, 207
 down-regulation protocol, 191
 flare protocol, 191, 192
 injections, 186–187, 193–196, **194,** 196, 198, 261–270
 intramuscular injections (muscle, IM), 186–187, 193, **194,** 195, 196
 intrauterine insemination (IUI), 186, 187, 189, 190, 191
 in vitro fertilization (IVF), 186, 187, 189, 190, 191–193
 protocols for in vitro fertilization (IVF), 191–193
 side effects, 187, 189, 192, 193, 196–197
 subcutaneous injections (skin, sub-Q), 186–187, **194,** 195–196, 196
 tips for injections, 194, **194,** 195, 197, 198, 261–270
 training, 197–199
Cycle day 2 (CD2), 192, 207

Cycle day 3 (CD3), 200–201, 207–208
Cycle day 7/9 (CD7/9), 208
Cycle paperwork, having, 181
Cycles performed by clinics, 50
Cystic fibrosis, 102
Cysts, 71–72
Cytogenic analysis, 58
Cytokines, 63–64, 95
Cytoplasm transfer, 92

Day-3 transfer, 224, 226
Day-5 transfer, 224, 225, 226, 227
D & C. *See* Dilation and curettage
Decisions about options, 117–148. *See also* Adoption; Stress management
 child-free living, 127–128, 279
 costs and, 118–119
 cryopreserving (freezing) of embryos, 146
 dietary changes, 126, 127
 egg donation, 128–131
 embryo donation, 131–132, 146, 279
 gamete intrafallopian transfer (GIFT), 137–140, 143, 144
 insurance and, 120, 132, 133
 intrauterine insemination (IUI), 132–134, 135, 146
 in vitro fertilization (IVF), 117, 134–137, 146
 lifestyle changes, 126
 medicated intrauterine insemination (IUI), 133
 mind-body work, 126, 278–279
 mistakes, avoiding, 118, 147, 180–181
 multiple birth risk, 144–146, 226, 227, 239
 natural cycle in vitro fertilization, 139–140
 natural intrauterine insemination (IUI), 133
 needles and, 118
 ovarian hyperstimulation syndrome (OHSS), 146–147
 plan for, 118, 147–148
 preeclampsia (high blood pressure), 144–145
 preimplantation genetic diagnosis (PGD), 58–59, 107, 140–141
 resources for, 278–279
 risks to consider, 144–147
 sperm donation, 128–131
 surrogates and gestational care, 141–143
 terminating treatment, 247–252
 third-party parenting, 141–143
 zygote intrafallopian transfer (ZIFT), 143–144
Deductible, insurance, 166, 167
Definition of success, clinics, 48–50
Denial of infertility, 3–4, 6

Denial of insurance claim, 165
Diagnosis, 73–98
    acquired blood-clotting disorder, 93
    "advanced maternal age," 4, 91, 97, 140
    alternative (holistic) therapies, 98, 125–127,
        278–279
    antiphospholipid antibodies (APA), 61–62, 93
    baby-killing cells, 60, 63–64, 95–97
    birth control pills (BCPs) for endometriosis,
        76
    blood-clotting disorders (thrombophilias), 12,
        60–61, 93–94
    "chocolate cyst" (endometrioma), 75
    Clomid challenge test, 90, 91
    cryomyolysis, 82
    cytokines, 63–64, 95
    cytoplasm transfer, 92
    dietary changes, 77, 86–87, 92
    donor eggs, 92
    ectopic pregnancy, 78
    education about, advocacy, 182
    egg quality, 56–57, 87, 88–92, 212–213
    endometrial biopsy, 65–67, 83
    endometriomas (hemorrhagic cysts), 75
    endometriosis, 4–5, 13–14, 71–72, 73–77
    estradiol (E2), 56–57, 88, 89–91
    fallopian tube problems, 3, 4, 5, 6, 67–70,
        74, 75, 77–80
    fibroids, 71–72, 80–82
    follicle-stimulating hormone (FSH), 56–57,
        88–89, 90–91
    genetic origins of endometriosis, 74
    heparin (Lovenox), 12, 15–16, 93–94
    high FSH, 88–92
    HLA compatibility, 63, 95–97
    hormone therapy for fibroids, 82
    hydrosalpinx, 79
    hysterectomy, 81–82
    immune problems, 12, 59–64, 93–97
    inherited blood-clotting disorder, 93
    insulin resistant, 86
    intravenous immunoglobulin or
        gammaglobulin (IVIG/IVGG), 19–20, 94,
        95–96
    in vitro fertilization (IVF) failure, 93–97
    laparoscopy, 4, 13, 71–72, 76, 78
    luteal phase defect (LPD), 65, 83–84
    lymphocyte immune therapy (LIT), 95, 96–
        97
    microsurgery, 78–79
    MTHFR mutation, 12, 13, 16, 61, 93
    myolysis, 82
    myomectomy, 82
    natural killer (NK) cells, 63, 95
    ovarian cysts, 4, 13, 75
    ovarian drilling, 87
    ovarian failure, 88–92
    ovaries, damaged, 74
    ovulation, 2–3, 4, 56, 57, 84–87
    polycystic ovarian syndrome (PCOS), 57, 84–
        87
    poor responders, 88–92
    premature ovarian failure (POF), 88–92
    progesterone support for luteal phase defect
        (LPD), 83
    recurrent pregnancy loss, 58–64, 93–97
    resected fallopian tube (reanastomosed), 79
    resources for, 276–277
    retrograde menstruation, 73–74
    tubal ligation repair, 79
    tubal microsurgery, 78
    "unexplained infertility," 97–98
    uterine artery embolization, 82
    uterine polyps or fibroids, 4, 13, 70–71, 81–
        82
    wedge resection, 87
Dietary changes
    decisions about options and, 126, 127
    Elizabeth Swire Falker's story, 13–14
    endometriosis, 77
    high FSH, 92
    male-factor infertility, 99
    polycystic ovarian syndrome (PCOS), 86–87
Dilation and curettage (D & C)
    blood tests, 58, 59, 64
    Elizabeth Swire Falker's story, 15, 19
    success of cycle, 243–244
Dividing (cleaving) of embryos, 223, 272
Doctor, finding, 5, 7. See also Reproductive
        endocrinologist (RE), finding
Domar, Alice, 126
Domestic adoption, 119, 121
Donated drugs, 177
Donor eggs, 92
Donor insemination, 105
Donor sperm, 9–10, 130
Dosage factors, medications, 190, 191
Down-regulation protocol, 191
Downtime between cycles, 245

E2. See Estradiol
Ectopic pregnancy, 78
Educating comment-maker, 155–156
Education about diagnosis, 182

Egg donation, 128–131
Egg management importance, 41
Egg quality vs. quantity, 56–57, 87, 88–92, 212–213
Egg retrieval calculation, clinics, 49
Eggs (number of) recruited for IVF, 46
E-mail option for responding to patient, 40
Embryo, implantation by, 11–12
Embryo donation, 131–132, 146, 279
Embryo and IVF, 228–230
Embryologists, 41, 42, 43
Embryology lab, 42, 43
Embryo quality, 223–227
Embryo toxicity assay (ETA), 64
Embryo transfer
  beginning treatment, 203, 222–223, 228–230
  clinic policies, 43
  frozen embryo transfers (FETs), 15–16, 17, 44, 230–233
Employer, negotiating with, 177
Employer-sponsored flexible spending accounts, 175
End of infertility, reaching (Rule #3), 28–29
Endometrial biopsy, 65–67, 83
Endometriomas (hemorrhagic cysts), 75
Endometriosis, 4–5, 13–14, 71–72, 73–77
Enemies at clinic, avoiding making, 183
Entertainment for stress management, 218–219
EOB (explanation of benefits), 166
Epididymis problems, 101–102
Estradiol (E2)
  blood test, 56–57, 88, 89–91
  monitoring, 209–211, 212, 214, 215
Estrogen, 11, 191
ETA (embryo toxicity assay), 64
Etingin, Orli, 12, 15–16, 19, 20
Exclusions of insurance policies, 162–163
Expectations, 209
Explanation of benefits (EOB), 166
Explanations by doctors, 35, 39

Facilitator adoption, 119, 125
Failed cycles, 222, 242
Failure, feelings of, 17
Falker, Elizabeth Swire, 1–22. *See also* Infertility
  acupuncture, 11
  adoption, xiii, xviii, xxi, 1, 19, 20 21
  "advanced maternal age," 4
  assisted reproductive technologies (ART), xxi, 7
  basal body temperature (BBT), 1–2

beta HCG level, 12, 14, 15
blood-clotting disorders (thrombophilias), 12
career decisions, 6–7, 8
Center for Reproductive Medicine and Infertility (CRMI), 5, 7, 11, 17–18
denial, 3–4, 6
dietary changes, 13–14
dilation and curettage (D & C), 15, 19
doctor, finding best possible, 5, 7
donor sperm, 9–10
embryos, implantation by, 11–12
endometriosis, 4–5, 13–14
failure, feelings of, 17
fallopian tubes, blocked, 3, 4, 5, 6
fertility drugs, 6
frozen embryo transfers (FETs), 15–16, 17
heparin (Lovenox) injections, 12, 15–16
home pregnancy tests (HPTs), 4
hyperhomocysteinemia, 12
hysterosalpinogram (HSG), 3, 6, 13
hysteroscopy, 7
immune issue, 12
implantation by embryos, 11–12
insurance, help with, 8
intracytoplasmic sperm injection (ICSI), 9, 10
intrauterine insemination (IUI), xxi, 6, 7, 8, 10, 109
intravenous immunoglobulin or gammaglobulin (IVIG/IVGG), 19–20
in vitro fertilization (IVF), xxi, 5–6, 7, 8, 9, 10–14, 16–20, 24
Kruger analysis, 8–9, 10
lactation, inducing, 21
laparoscopy, 4, 13
Lovenox injections, 16, 269–270
luteal phase of menstrual cycle, 11, 12
male-factor infertility, 3–4, 9–10
marriage counseling, 2
miscarriages, 15, 20, 21
motherhood, xix–xx, 1
MTHFR gene, 12, 13, 16
OB-GYN, 1, 2, 3, 4
organic diet, 14
ovarian cysts, 4, 13
ovarian hyperstimulation syndrome (OHSS), 20
ovulation, 2 3, 4
ovulation induction, 6
ovulation predictor kit (OPK), 3
personal side of a doctor and, 5
positive pregnancy BBT mark, 4

pregnancies, 14–15, 18
progesterone levels, 11
reproductive endocrinologist (RE), 2, 5, 7
second opinions, 16
sperm morphology, 9–10
stress, 6–7
uterine polyps or fibroids, 4, 13
weight gain from in vitro fertilization (IVF), 11
Fallopian tubes, blocked, 3, 4, 5, 6, 67–70, 74, 75, 77–80
Family-building options. *See* Decisions about options
Family Fee Plan, 175, 279
Family members and infertility, xv–xvi. *See also* Friends and family
Female vs. male REs, 36–37
*Fertility and Sterility*, 94, 216, 218
Fertility clinic, finding best, 5, 7. *See also* Reproductive endocrinologist (RE), finding
Fertility drugs, 6
"Fertility Inc.: Clinics Race to Lure Clients" (Kolata), 47
Fertinex, **188**
FETs (frozen embryo transfers), 15–16, 17, 44, 230–233
Fibroids, 71–72, 80–82
Financial aspects of infertility, 160–179. *See also* Costs; Insurance; Shared-risk programs
costs of infertility workup, 160–161
credit cards for, 175
donated drugs, 177
employer-sponsored flexible spending accounts, 175
Family Fee Plan, 175, 279
flexible spending accounts, employer-sponsored, 175
401(k) plans for, 175
home equity loan for, 175
Internet drug caution, 177–178
limits of financial exposure, 176
loans, low-interest, 174–175
low-interest loans, 174–175
medication, paying for, 177–178
on-line pharmacy, 178, 279–280
package deals, 174
planning for, 201
research study by drug company, 177
resources for, 279–280
retirement plans for, 175

Flare protocol, 191, 192
Flexibility for adoption, 121
Flexible spending accounts, employer-sponsored, 175
Follicle development, 209, 212, 214
Follicle-stimulating hormone (FSH)
diagnosis and, 56–57, 88–89, 90–91
medications and, 186–191, **188**
sperm analysis, 102
Follistim, **188,** 189, 190, 196, 197
Foster care adoption, 125
401(k) plans for infertility payment, 175
Fragmentation, 223–224
Freezing eggs criteria, 44
Freezing. *See* Cryopreserving
Friends and family, 149–159
agreeing with comment-maker, 154–155
baby showers, 156–157
bosses, caution, 153
categories of, 151–153
condescending suggestions, 154
confronting comment-maker, 155–156
educating comment-maker, 155–156
honesty for, 156, 159
hope and inspiration from, 158–159
human resources department, caution, 153
insensitive comments, coping, 149–150, 153–156
lying for, 156
networking, 151
opinionated people, 154
secrecy, backfiring, 149–151
social obligations, coping, 156–157
support from, xvi, 113–116, 149, 152–153, 219
thoughtless comments, 154
what to say, 151–153
who to tell, 151–153
work obligations, coping with, 153, 156, 157–158, 178–179
Friends with children, xv
Frozen embryo transfers (FETs), 15–16, 17, 44, 230–233
FSH. *See* Follicle-stimulating hormone

GA (prothrombin gene mutation 20210), 61
Gamete intrafallopian transfer (GIFT), 137–140, 143, 144
Gender of baby and adoption, 121
Gene mutations, sperm analysis, 102
Genetic karyotyping, 58–59, 110

Genetic origins of endometriosis, 74

Gestational care and surrogates, 141–143

GIFT (gamete intrafallopian transfer), 137–140, 143, 144

Gladney Center for Adoption, 20

Glucophage (metformin), 86, 87

Gonal-F, **188,** 189, 190, 193, 196

Gray area, normal vs. abnormal, 104–105

Gut instinct, trusting, 38

Gynecologists (GYNs), 30

Health insurance claim form (HICF), 164–167. *See also* Insurance

Health issues and male-factor infertility, 106

Hell of infertility, xx–xxii

Hemorrhagic cysts (endometriomas), 75

Heparin (Lovenox), 12, 15–16, 93–94

HICF (health insurance claim form), 164–167. *See also* Insurance

High blood pressure (preeclampsia), 144–145

High FSH, 88–92

HLA (human leukocyte antigens), 63, 95–97

Holistic (alternative) therapies, 98, 125–127, 278–279

Home equity loan for infertility payment, 175

Homeopathy treatments, 127

Home pregnancy tests (HPTs), 4, 236–237, 238

Honesty about infertility, 156, 159

Hope from friends, 158–159

Hormonal system, 65–67

Hormone imbalance, sperm analysis, 102

Hormone therapy for fibroids, 82

Horrible experience for everyone (Rule #2), 25–28, 29

HPTs (home pregnancy tests), 4, 236–237, 238

HSG (hysterosalpinogram), 3, 6, 13, 67–69

Human chorionic gonadotropin (HCG)
  beginning treatment, 207, 208, 212, 214–215
  beta HCG test, 12, 14, 15, 236, 237–240, **240**
  medications, **188,** 190, 195

Human leukocyte antigens (HLA), 63, 95–97

Human resources department, caution, 153

Humegon, **188**

Hydrosalpinx, 79

Hyperhomocysteinemia, 12, 61

Hypnosis, 217

Hypospadia, 109

Hysterectomy, 81–82

Hysterosalpinogram (HSG), 3, 6, 13, 67–69

Hysteroscopy, 7, 70–71, 81

ICSI. *See* Intracytoplasmic sperm injection

Identical twins and ICSI, 106

IM (intramuscular injections), 186–187, 193, **194,** 195, 196

Immune problems, 12, 59–64, 93–97

Implantation, 11–12, 234

Implantation spotting, 233–234

Inducing lactation, 21

Infertility, xv–xxii. *See also* Advocacy; Beginning treatment; Blood tests; Clinic evaluation; Cycle, understanding your; Decisions about options; Diagnosis; Falker, Elizabeth Swire; Financial aspects of infertility; Friends and family; Insurance; Invasive tests; Male-factor infertility; Monitoring treatment; Reproductive endocrinologist (RE), finding; Shared-risk programs; Success of cycle; Surviving infertility roller coaster; Urologists and sperm analyses
  benefits of, xviii–xix, 253–254
  family members and, xv–xvi
  friends with children and, xv
  hell of, xx–xxii
  learning about yourself from, xviii–xix, xx, 253–254
  life changes from, xix–xx, 253–254
  obsessing about having a baby, xvii–xviii
  "platinum" infertility status, xviii
  pregnant friends and, xv, xvi
  self-knowledge from, xviii–xix, xx, 253–254
  sex life, xvii
  support for, xvi, 113–116, 149, 152–153, 219
  understanding of, xv–xvii

Inflated success, clinics, 49, 50, 51

Inherited blood-clotting disorder, 93

Inherited thrombophilias, 60–61

Injections, 186–187, 193–196, **194,** 196, 198, 261–270

Insensitive comments, coping with, 149–150, 153–156

Insulin resistance, 86

Insurance, 162–168. *See also* Financial aspects of infertility
  checklist, 167–168
  Consolidated Omnibus Budget Reconciliation Act (COBRA), 176
  decisions about options and, 120, 132, 133
  deductible, 166, 167
  denial of claim, fighting, 165
  employer, negotiating with, 177

exclusions of policies, 162–163
explanation of benefits (EOB), 166
health insurance claim form (HICF), 164–167
help with insurance, 8, 163–164
limitations of policies, 162–163
loss of insurance coverage, 176–177
mail-order drug service, 178
out-of-pocket deductible, 166
precertification requirements, 163
reproductive endocrinologists (REs) and, 37–38, 52
self-employment and, 176
spouse's plan, 177
state laws for, 162
usual and customary rate (UCR), 166, 167
IntegraMed, 169, 173, 279
International adoption, 119, 121, 124
Internet drug caution, 177–178
Internet for REs, 33–34
Interpretation problems of semen analyses, 104
Interview questions for REs, 31, 32, 34, 38–48, 257–259
Intracytoplasmic sperm injection (ICSI), 271
    birth defects and, 106–107
    decisions about options, 136
    Elizabeth Swire Falker's story, 9, 10
    identical twins and, 106
    male-factor infertility, 99, 100, 102, 103, 105, 106–107, 108
    reproductive endocrinologists (REs) and, 44, 47
    rescue intracytoplasmic sperm injection, 47, 107
Intramuscular injections (muscle, IM), 186–187, 193, **194**, 195, 196
Intrauterine insemination (IUI)
    beginning treatment, 201–202, 206, 219–220
    decisions about options, 132–134, 135, 146
    Elizabeth Swire Falker's story, xxi, 6, 7, 8, 10, 109
    understanding cycle, 186, 187, 189, 190, 191
Intravenous immunoglobulin or gammaglobulin (IVIG/IVGG), 19–20, 94, 95–96
Invasive tests, 64–72. See also Blood tests
    adhesions, 71–72
    cysts, 71–72
    endometrial biopsy, 65–67, 83
    endometriosis, 4–5, 13–14, 71–72, 73–77
    fallopian tubes, 3, 4, 5, 6, 67–70, 74, 75, 77–80

fibroids, 71–72, 80–82
    hormonal system, 65–67
    hysterosalpinogram (HSG), 3, 6, 13, 67–69
    hysteroscopy, 70–71, 81
    laparoscopy, 4, 13, 71–72, 76, 78
    luteal phase defect (LPD), 65, 83–84
    saline sonogram/HSG, 69–70
    TLC after, 66
    tubal catheterization (transversal cannulation), 68
    uterine cavity, 67–70
    uterine lining, 65–67, 215
    uterine polyps or fibroids, 4, 13, 70–71, 81–82
In vitro fertilization (IVF)
    beginning treatment, 201, 202–203, 206, 220–223
    decisions about options, 117, 134–137, 146
    Elizabeth Swire Falker's story, xxi, 5–6, 7, 8, 9, 10–14, 16–20, 24
    embryo transfer and, 228–230
    failure, 58–64, 93–97
    success rates, 50–51
    understanding cycle, 186, 187, 189, 190, 191–193
IUI. See Intrauterine insemination
IVF. See In vitro fertilization
IVIG/IVGG (intravenous immunoglobulin or gammaglobulin), 19–20, 94, 95–96

Kallman's syndrome, 102
Klinefelter's syndrome, 102
Kolata, Gina, 47
Kruger analysis, 8–9, 10, 103, 104

Lab competence. See Clinic evaluation
Lab differences and sperm analysis, 104
Lab specific tests, 56–57
Lactation, inducing, 21
Laparoscopy, 4, 13, 71–72, 76, 78
"Last resort" clinics, 52
Layers of infertility (Rule #3), 28–29
Learning about yourself from infertility, xviii–xix, xx, 253–254
Leiden factor V mutation R560Q, 61
LH. See Luteinizing hormone
Life changes from infertility, xix–xx, 253–254
Lifestyle changes and options, 126
Lifestyle changes for male-factor infertility, 99
Limitations of insurance, 162–163
Limits of financial exposure, 176

List of priorities (your), developing, 31–32, 34, 35–40
LIT (lymphocyte immune therapy), 95, 96–97
Live-birth rates, 49
Living through the cycle. *See* Beginning treatment
Loans, low-interest, 174–175
Location of clinic, 37, 53–54
Loss of insurance coverage, 176–177
Lovenox (heparin), 12, 15–16, 93–94
Lovenox injections, 16, 93–94, 269–270
Low-interest loans, 174–175
LPD (luteal phase defect), 65, 83–84
Lupron, 76, 82, **188,** 190, 191–192
Lupuslike anticoagulant antibodies, 61, 62
Luteal phase defect (LPD), 65, 83–84
Luteal phase of menstrual cycle, 11, 12
Luteinizing hormone (LH)
    diagnosis and, 56–57, 215
    medications and, 189
Lying about infertility, 156
Lymphocyte immune therapy (LIT), 95, 96–97

Mail-order drug service, 178
Male-factor infertility, 99–116. *See also*
    Intracytoplasmic sperm injection (ICSI);
    Urologists and sperm analyses
    anatomical issues, 107–109
    birth defects and ICSI, 106–107
    cryopreserving (freezing) of sperm, 113
    dietary changes for, 99
    donor sperm, 9–10, 130
    Elizabeth Swire Falker's story, 3–4, 9–10
    genetic karyotyping, 58–59, 110
    hypospadia, 109
    identical twins and ICSI, 106
    lifestyle changes for, 99
    microsurgical epididymal sperm aspiration (MESA), 111, 112
    multiple standard biopsy, 112
    nonobstructive azoospermia, 112
    obstructive azoospermia, 111–112
    percutaneous biopsy of the testis (PercBiopsy), 111–112
    percutaneous epididymal sperm aspiration (PESA), 111
    preimplantation genetic diagnosis (PGD), 58–59, 107, 140–141
    reproductive endocrinologists (REs), 30–31
    reproductive tract blockages, 101, 109
    rescue intracytoplasmic sperm injection (ICSI), 47, 107

resources for, 277
retrograde ejaculation, 109
statistics on, 99
supporting the infertile man, 113–116
surgery for removal of sperm, 110–113
testicular fine needle aspiration (TFNA), 111, 112
testicular sperm extraction (TESA), 112, 113
treatability of, 99–100
varicoceles, 101, 102, 105, 107–108
vas deferens malformation (CAV), 102, 108–109
Male vs. female REs, 36–37
Marketing tactics of clinics, 47–48
Marriage counseling, 2
Massage, 218
Medical history, urologists, 101
Medical records
    knowledge of, 181
    sending to doctor in advance, 38
Medicated IUI, 133
Medications, 186–191. *See also* Cycle, understanding your
    Antagon, **188,** 190, 192
    birth control pills (BCPs), 76, 192–193
    Climara, **188**
    Clomid, 26, 69, 83, 133, 187, **188,** 189, 190, 196
    controlled ovarian hyperstimulation, 186
    dosage factors, 190, 191
    estrogen, 11, 191
    Fertinex, **188**
    follicle-stimulating hormone (FSH, stims), 186–191, **188**
    follicle stimulating hormone (FSH) in, 189
    Follistim, **188,** 189, 190, 196, 197
    Gonal-F, **188,** 189, 190, 193, 196
    heparin (Lovenox), 12, 15–16, 93–94
    human chorionic gonadotropin (HCG), **188,** 190, 195
    Humegon, **188**
    Lovenox injections, 16, 93–94, 269–270
    Lupron, 76, 82, **188,** 190, 191–192
    luteinizing hormone (LH) in, 189
    menstrual cycle suppressions, 190
    Metrodin, **188**
    paying for, 177–178
    Pergonal, **188,** 189, 193, 195, 196
    progesterone, 83, **188,** 190–191, 234
    progesterone in oil (PIO), **188,** 191, 234, 269
    Propofol, 221

recombinant follicle stimulating hormone (FSH), 189
Repronex, **188,** 189, 190, 193
Serophene, **188**
side effects, 187, 189, 192, 193, 196–197
Synarel, 76, 82, **188,** 190, 191, 192
Meditation, 126, 217
Menstrual cycle suppressions, 190
Menstrual/ovulation cycle, 255–257
MESA (microsurgical epididymal sperm aspiration), 111, 112
Metformin (Glucophage), 86, 87
Metrodin, **188**
Microsurgery, 78–79
Microsurgical epididymal sperm aspiration (MESA), 111, 112
Mind-body work, 126, 278–279
Miscarriages, 15, 20, 21, 242, 243–244
Mistakes, preventing, 118, 147, 180–181
Mittelschmerz (midcycle pain), 206
Money-back-guarantee programs, 168. *See also* Shared-risk programs
Monitoring treatment, 208–216. *See also* Beginning treatment; Stress management
  canceling cycle, 211
  "coasting," 210
  comparisons, avoiding, 209
  egg quality vs. quantity, 56–57, 87, 88–92, 212–213
  estradiol (E2), 209–211, 212, 214, 215
  expectations and, 209
  follicle development, 209, 212, 214
  human chorionic gonadotropin (HCG), **188,** 190, 195, 207, 208, 212, 214–215
  luteinizing hormone (LH), 56–57, 215
  ovarian hyperstimulation syndrome (OHSS), 20, 46, 146–147, 210–211
  pacing yourself, 216
  quality of egg vs. quantity, 56–57, 87, 88–92, 212–213
  slow and steady wins, 213–215
  stims, responding to, 209–212
  triple stripe uterine lining, 215
  uterine lining, 65–67, 215
Morphology of sperm, 9–10, 103, 104, 105
Motherhood, xix–xx, 1
Mother's background and adoption, 121
Motility of sperm, 103, 104, 105
MTHFR gene, 12, 13, 16, 61, 93
Multiple births, 144–146, 226, 227, 239
Multiple standard biopsy, 112

Muscle (intramuscular) injections (IM), 186–187, 193, **194,** 195, 196
Myolysis, 82
Myomectomy, 82

National Institute of Child Health and Human Development Reproductive Medicine Network (NIH), 104
Natural cycle IVF, 139–140
Natural IUI, 133
Natural killer (NK) cells, 63, 95
Naturopathic treatment, 126–127
Needles, decisions about options, 118
Needs (your), determining, 31–32, 34, 35–40
Negative beta, 242–243
Networking, 151
New York Presbyterian Hospital, Cornell Medical Center, 12
NK (natural killer) cells, 63, 95
Nonobstructive azoospermia, 112
No-nonsense doctors, 35
Number of procedures performed weekly/yearly, 43, 44, 45

OB-GYN, 1, 2, 3, 4, 30
Obsessing about having a baby, xvii–xviii
Obstructive azoospermia, 111–112
O'Donnell, Rosie, 120
OHSS (ovarian hyperstimulation syndrome), 20, 46, 146–147, 210–211
Older couples and adoption, 124
On-line pharmacy, 178, 279–280
Oocyte retrieval, 203, 220–222
Open adoption, 121–122, 129
Opinionated people, 154
OPK (ovulation predictor kit), 3
Opt-out provision, shared-risk programs, 173–174
Organic diet, 14
Organizations for referrals, 32–33
Out-of-pocket deductible, 166
Ovarian cysts, 4, 13, 75
Ovarian drilling, 87
Ovarian failure, 88–92
Ovarian hyperstimulation syndrome (OHSS), 20, 46, 146–147, 210–211
Ovaries, damaged, 74
Ovulation, 2–3, 4, 56, 57, 84–87
Ovulation induction, 6
Ovulation predictor kit (OPK), 3

Pacing yourself, 216

Package deals, 174

Parenting right of birth mother, 123

Patient coordinators, 202

PCOS (polycystic ovarian syndrome), 57, 84–87

Peeling the onion of infertility (Rule #3), 28–29

Percutaneous biopsy of the testis (PercBiopsy), 111–112

Percutaneous epididymal sperm aspiration (PESA), 111

Pergonal, **188,** 189, 193, 195, 196

Personal side of doctor, 5, 31–32

Per-transfer calculation, clinics, 49

PESA (percutaneous epididymal sperm aspiration), 111

PGD (preimplantation genetic diagnosis), 58–59, 107, 140–141

Phone calls returned by doctor/nurse, 36, 40

Physical exam, urologists, 101

PIO (progesterone in oil), **188,** 191, 234, 269

Plan for treatment, 118, 147–148

"Platinum" infertility status, xviii

POF (premature ovarian failure), 88–92

Polycystic ovarian syndrome (PCOS), 57, 84–87

Poor responders, 88–92

Positive pregnancy BBT mark, 4

Precertification requirements of insurance, 163

Prednisone for blood clotting disorders, 94

Preeclampsia (high blood pressure), 144–145

Pregnancy
    clinic rates, 48
    Elizabeth Swire Falker's story, 14–15, 18
    friends, xv, xvi
    shared-risk programs and, 170–171
    signs, 233–234
    stress management for, 216
    success of cycle, 240–242
    test, 235

"Pregnancy worthy" embryos, 231

Preimplantation genetic diagnosis (PGD), 58–59, 107, 140–141

Premature ovarian failure (POF), 88–92

Prescreened lists of physicians, 32–33

Private attorney adoption, 119, 121, 122–124

Procedures available at clinic, 44

Progesterone, 83, **188,** 190–191, 234

Progesterone for LPD, 83

Progesterone in oil (PIO), **188,** 191, 234, 269

Progesterone levels, 11

Prognosis, 47

Program FET, 231–232

Prolactin blood test, 57

Propofol, 221

Prostate problems, 102

Protein C or S abnormalities, 61

Prothrombin gene mutation 20210 (GA), 61

Protocols for IVF, 191–193

Protocols used by REs, 47

Published articles by REs, 42

Quacks, 31

Quality of egg vs. quantity, 56–57, 87, 88–92, 212–213

Questions for REs, 31, 32, 34, 38–48, 257–259

RE. *See* Reproductive endocrinologist

Reanastomosed (resected fallopian tube), 79

Recombinant FSH, 189

Recurrent pregnancy loss, 58–64, 93–97

Referrals
    for adoption, 125
    for reproductive endocrinologists (REs), 32–33, 47
    for urologists, 100

Relaxation therapy, 217

Relinquishment laws, 123

Reproductive endocrinologist (RE), finding, 30–54. *See also* Clinic evaluation; Success rates of clinics
    aggressiveness of, 46–47
    assisted hatching, 44, 47, 227
    board certification, 30, 42
    business of reproductive medicine, 31, 34, 47, 182
    "Buyer beware," 34
    cancellation criteria for cycle, 46
    compassionate doctors, 32, 35
    eggs (number of) recruited for in vitro fertilization (IVF), 46
    Elizabeth Swire Falker's story, 2, 5, 7
    E-mail option for response, 40
    explanations by doctors, 35, 39
    female vs. male, 36–37
    gut instinct, trusting, 38
    insurance and, 37–38, 52
    Internet for, 33–34
    interview questions, 31, 32, 34, 38–48, 257–259
    intracytoplasmic sperm injection (ICSI), 44, 47
    location, convenience of, 37, 53–54

male-factor infertility, 30–31
male vs. female, 36–37
marketing tactics, 47–48
medical records, in advance, 38
needs (your), determining, 31–32, 34, 35–40
no-nonsense doctors, 35
OB-GYN vs., 1, 2, 3, 4, 30
organizations for referrals, 32–33
ovarian hyperstimulation syndrome (OHSS) percentage, 46
personal side of, 5, 31–32
phone calls returned by, 36, 40
prescreened lists of, 32–33
prognosis, 47
protocols used by, 47
published articles by, 42
quacks, 31
question asking by patients, 39
referrals for, 32–33, 47
rescue intracytoplasmic sperm injection (ICSI), 47, 107
resources for, 275–276
start of treatment recommendations, 46
state-of-the art practice of, 31, 32, 37, 52
techniques (new) developed by, 42
time allocated to appointments, 39
urologists, 30–31, 32
waiting rooms, 35–36
Web sites for, 33–34
Reproductive immunophenotype test (RIP), 63
Reproductive tract blockages, male, 101, 109
Repronex, **188,** 189, 190, 193
Reputation of agencies, 125
Rescue ICSI, 47, 107
Research-based medical center, 42
Research study sponsored by drug company, 177
Resected fallopian tube (reanastomosed), 79
RESOLVE, 32, 100, 141, 219
Resources for infertility, 275–280
Resting during IVF, 203
Retirement plans for infertility payment, 175
Retrieval (oocyte retrieval), 203, 220–222
Retrograde ejaculation, 109
Retrograde menstruation, 73–74
Returning phone calls by doctor, 36, 40
RIP (reproductive immunophenotype test), 63
Risk factors for male-factor infertility, 101
Risks
  of adoption, 123, 125, 132
  of decisions about options, 144–147
  of medications, 187, 189, 192, 193, 196–197
  of shared-risk programs, 171–173

Saline sonogram/HSG, 69–70
Same-sex couples and adoption, 124
Scheduling cycle, 200–204
Second opinions, 16
Secrecy about infertility, 149–151
Selective reduction, 239
Self-employment and insurance, 176
Self-hypnosis, 217
Self-knowledge from infertility, xviii–xix, xx, 253–254
Semen count, 103, 104, 105
Seminal fluid pH, 103
Semiopen adoption, 121, 122
Sensitivity of body, 206–207
Serophene, **188**
Serum progesterone blood test, 56
Sex life, xvii
Sexual history, urologists, 101
Shared-risk programs, 168–174. See also Financial aspects of infertility
  age and, 169, 170
  aggressiveness of, 173
  comparisons of, 171–173
  criteria for, 169–170
  IntegraMed, 169, 173, 279
  money-back-guarantee programs, 168
  opt-out provision, 173–174
  pregnancy and, 170–171
  risks of, 171–173
  success definitions, 173
Shots. See Injections
Side effects of medications, 187, 189, 192, 193, 196–197
Skin (subcutaneous) injections (sub-Q), 186–187, **194,** 195–196, 196
Slow and steady wins, 213–215
Small vs. big clinics, 40–41
Social obligations, coping, 156–157
Society for Assisted Reproductive Technologies (SART), 48
SPA (sperm penetration assay), 105
Sperm analyses. See Urologists and sperm analyses
Sperm density, 103, 104, 105
Sperm donation, 128–131
Sperm management of clinic, 41
Sperm morphology, 9–10, 103, 104, 105
Sperm motility, 103, 104, 105
Sperm needed for pregnancy, 100, 105

Sperm penetration assay (SPA), 105
Spielberg, Steven, 120
Spouse's insurance plan, 177
Standing up for yourself, 183–184
Starting with a clean slate (Rule #1), 23–25, 29
Start of treatment recommendations, 46
State laws for insurance coverage, 162
State-of-the art practice, 31, 32, 37, 52
Stein-Leventhal Syndrome (PCOS), 57, 84–87
Steps of treatment, knowing, 181–182
Stims, responding to, 209–212
Stims phase and OHSS, 147
Stress management, 216–219. *See also* Beginning
    treatment
  acupuncture, 11, 92, 126, 127, 217–218
  alternative (holistic) therapies, 98, 125–127,
    278–279
  biofeedback techniques, 126
  Elizabeth Swire Falker's story, 6–7
  entertainment for, 218–219
  hypnosis for, 217
  infertility treatment and, 202, 203–204, 207
  massage for, 218
  meditation for, 126, 217
  pregnancy chances and, 216
  relaxation therapy for, 217
  self-hypnosis for, 217
  support groups for, 219
  talking for, 219
  visualization for, 217
  yoga for, 218
Stress-reduction techniques, 126
Subcutaneous injections (skin, sub-Q), 186–187,
    **194,** 195–196, 196
Success definitions of shared-risk programs, 173
Success of cycle, 236–246. *See also* Decisions
    about options
  beta HCG test, 12, 14, 15, 236, 237–240,
    **240**
  celebrating pregnancy, 241–242
  dilation and curettage (D & C), 243–244
  downtime between cycles, 245
  failed cycles, 222, 242
  home pregnancy tests (HPTs), 4, 236–237,
    238
  miscarriages, 15, 20, 21, 242, 243–244
  multiples, 239
  negative beta, 242–243
  pregnancy, 240–242
  resources for, 280
  selective reduction, 239
  survivor's guilt, 241

Success rates of clinics, 47–52. *See also* Clinic
    evaluation; Reproductive endocrinologist
    (RE), finding
  admission policies and, 51–52
  audited statistics, 48
  blastocyst transfer rates, 51
  chemical pregnancy rates, 49, 50
  clinical pregnancy rates, 49, 50
  cycles (number) performed, 50
  definition of success, 48–50
  egg retrieval calculation, 49
  inflated success rates, 49, 50, 51
  interviewing doctors and, 34
  in vitro fertilization (IVF) rates, 50–51
  "last resort" clinics, 52
  live-birth rates, 49
  per-transfer calculation, 49
  pregnancy rate, 48
  statistics, 48–50, 259–261, **260**
  women cycling calculation, 49
  "world-famous" clinics, 52
Support for infertility, xvi, 113–116, 149, 152–
    153, 219
Surgery for removal of sperm, 110–113
Surrogates and gestational care, 141–143
Surviving infertility roller coaster, 23–29. *See*
    *also* Decisions about options; Infertility
  addictiveness of treatment, 247–248
  clean slate, starting with (Rule #1), 23–25,
    29
  end of infertility, reaching (Rule #3), 28–29
  horrible experience for everyone (Rule #2),
    25–28, 29
  peeling the onion of infertility (Rule #3), 28–
    29
  starting with a clean slate (Rule #1), 23–25,
    29
Survivor's guilt, 241
Synarel, 76, 82, **188,** 190, 191, 192
Syndrome O/X (PCOS), 57, 84–87

Talking for stress management, 219
Technical competence, evaluating, 40–45
Techniques developed by REs, 42
Terminating treatment, 247–252
TESA (testicular sperm extraction), 112, 113
Testicle problems, 101
Testicular fine needle aspiration (TFNA), 111,
    112
Testicular sperm extraction (TESA), 112, 113
Testing process, 55. *See also* Blood tests;
    Invasive tests

TFNA (testicular fine needle aspiration), 111, 112

Third-party parenting, 141–143

Thoughtless comments, 154

Thrombophilias (blood clotting disorders), 12, 60–61, 93–94

Time allocated to appointments, 39

TLC after invasive tests, 66

TNF (tumor necrosis factor), 63

Training for cycle, 197–199

Transrectal ultrasound procedure, 101

Transversal cannulation (tubal catheterization), 68

Triple stripe uterine lining, 215

Tubal catheterization (transversal cannulation), 68

Tubal ligation repair, 79

Tubal microsurgery, 78

Tumor necrosis factor (TNF), 63

Two-week wait, 229, 233–235

UCR (usual and customary rate), 166, 167

Understanding of infertility, xv–xvii. *See also* Infertility

"Unexplained infertility," 97–98

Urologists and sperm analyses, 100–106. *See also* Male-factor infertility

  azoospermia, 102, 111–113

  blood tests, 102

  cystic fibrosis, 102

  donor insemination, 105

  epididymis problems, 101–102

  finding best, 30–31, 32

  follicle stimulating hormone (FSH), 102

  gene mutations, 102

  gray area, normal vs. abnormal, 104–105

  health issues implicated by, 106

  hormone imbalance, 102

  interpretation problems, 104

  Kallman's syndrome, 102

  Klinefelter's syndrome, 102

  Kruger analysis, 8–9, 10, 103, 104

  lab differences and, 104

  medical history, 101

  morphology of sperm, 9–10, 103, 104, 105

  motility of sperm, 103, 104, 105

  physical exam, 101

  prostate problems, 102

  referrals for urologists, 100

  reproductive tract blockages, 101, 109

  risk factors for male-factor infertility, 101

  semen count, 103, 104, 105

  seminal fluid pH, 103

  sexual history, 101

  sperm needed for pregnancy, 100, 105

  sperm penetration assay (SPA), 105

  testicle problems, 101

  transrectal ultrasound procedure, 101

  varicoceles, 101, 102, 105, 107–108

  vas deferens malformation (CAV), 102, 108–109

  viscosity of fluid, 103

  World Health Organization (WHO) standards, 103, 104

  Y chromosome mutation, 102

Usual and customary rate (UCR), 166, 167

Uterine artery embolization, 82

Uterine cavity, 67–70

Uterine lining, 65–67, 215

Uterine polyps or fibroids, 4, 13, 70–71, 81–82

Varicoceles, 101, 102, 105, 107–108

Vas deferens malformation (CAV), 102, 108–109

Venting, avoiding, 183

Vials, preparing injection using, 265–269

Viscosity of fluid, sperm analysis, 103

Visualization, 217

Waiting rooms, 35–36

Wait list for cycle, 202

Wait time for adoption, 121

Web sites for REs, 33–34

Wedge resection, 87

Weight gain from IVF, 11

What to say about infertility, 151–153

Who to tell about infertility, 151–153

Winfrey, Oprah, 120

Women cycling calculation, clinics, 49

Work obligations, coping, 153, 156, 157–158, 178–179

"World-famous" clinics, 52

World Health Organization (WHO), 103, 104

Y chromosome mutation, 102

Yoga, 218

Zona pellucida (shell) of embryo, 223, 227

Zygote intrafallopian transfer (ZIFT), 143–144

**Elizabeth Swire Falker** spent seven years trying to conceive. She gave up her career as a lawyer when she found she couldn't struggle with infertility while working at a high-powered job. She now lives in Westchester County, New York, with her husband and their adopted son.